T0349377

SAS FITNESS TRAINING

AN ELITE WORKOUT PROGRAMME FOR YOUR BODY AND MIND

SAS AND SPECIAL FORCES

FITNESS TRAINING

AN ELITE WORKOUT PROGRAMME FOR YOUR BODY AND MIND

JOHN 'LOFTY' WISEMAN

amber
BOOKS

This revised Amber edition first published in 2024

First published in 1996 as *The SAS Personal Trainer*

Copyright © Amber Books Ltd 2024

Published by
Amber Books Ltd
United House
North Road
London N7 9DP
United Kingdom
www.amberbooks.co.uk
Facebook: amberbooks
YouTube: amberbooksltd
Instagram: amberbooksltd
X(Twitter): @amberbooks

ISBN 978-1-83886-453-8

Printed in China

All illustrations courtesy Amber Books Ltd.

Picture credits
Airsealand.Photos: 83, 88, 93, 99, 121
Allsport: 114, 120, 137
Amber Books: 20
Berghaus: 95
Dreamstime: 9 (Martinmark), 10 (peopleimages), 23 (Wavebreakmedia), 47 (Lunamarina), 82 (Dziewul), 84 (Sutthinon602), 109 (Martinmark), 112 (Kovop58)
Format: 31
Getty Images: 111 (David Ramos)
Sally & Richard Greenhill: 45
The Image Bank: 13, 61, 90, 108, 113
Impact Photos: 110, 115, 119
Rex Features: 49
Mark Shearman: 50, 51, 87, 97, 98
Shutterstock: 85 (Anton Watman)
YHA Adventures Shops Plc: 91

Contents

1 STRENGTH & ENDURANCE

CHAPTER ONE

The Importance of Being Fit

It has always seemed strange to me that people may lavish every attention on their cars, but more often than not neglect the most valuable possession they will ever have: their bodies. We cannot exchange our bodies, unlike our cars, for more recent models, but we can regularly service and fine-tune them, thus ensuring, illness aside, that they remain in good repair for the rest of our lives.

More importantly, the healthier we stay, the more we are likely to get out of life, allowing us to live life to the full. Maintaining good health also helps in avoiding illness and injuries. Fitness generates the confidence that will enable you to handle any situation.

Medical science has demonstrated that if we keep fit and try to maintain a healthy diet, we stand a better chance of living longer and surviving health hazards. In extreme situations, your level of fitness and overall health can make the difference between living and dying.

We are becoming more aware of the stress in our lives. Stress is something which concerns us all. The senior manager and the housewife will experience different types of stress, but the effect will be same. If you suffer from a poor appetite, interrupted sleep, feelings of unease or of not being in control of your life, or just a general lack of confidence, these fitness programmes will help you. Everyone can improve their lifestyle and get greater enjoyment by following a simple fitness programme.

Overall fitness can be broken down into three categories: suppleness, stamina and strength, and all three 'Ss' are targeted in the fitness programmes presented in this book. Younger people will be likely to place emphasis on strength and stamina, while older people may want to spend more time doing suppleness exercises. Nevertheless, a degree of flexibility is important for all of us to have. For example, freedom of movement and joint rotation is especially important in self-defence.

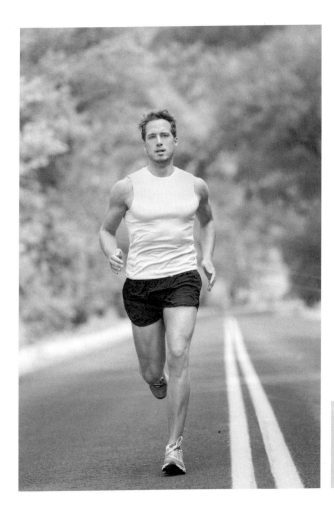

Following a fitness programme will go a long way to ensuring a healthier and more fulfilled life. Feeling fit gives you confidence to tackle whatever life may throw at you.

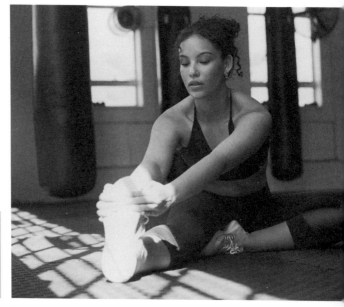

Warming up and stretching exercises are vitally important in preparing the body for a strenuous work-out. Without these, we risk nagging injuries to muscles and ligaments.

Speed and power depend upon a high degree of suppleness. If we begin every exercise programme with a gentle warm-up and a series of stretching exercises, blood starts to flow to the muscles and we help avoid the small muscle tears and strained ligaments caused by sudden explosive movements. Equally, after a vigorous exercise session we must cool down with a series of gentle exercises, thus allowing our bodies to return to normal.

BE CAREFUL: Too much exercise, too soon, can lead to injury. Begin slowly and build up speed and the number of times you repeat the exercise ('repetitions') gradually. If you have not exercised for some time, start by taking short walks. Start thinking 'fitness'. Get off the bus one stop before home. Use the stairs instead of taking the lift. Walk to the

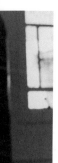

local shops instead of driving. Do a little exercise every day and you will soon experience the benefit. Do not be put off by the initial discomfort; it is always hard work when you begin. You will soon get into a routine and the aches will disappear as your fitness increases.

REMEMBER: If you start to experience chest-pains, pains shooting up the arms, prolonged breathlessness, sweating or headaches, see your doctor.

Special Training: Considerations for Women

The Olympics, modern athletics and military service were all devised by men for men. Women have had a long uphill struggle against male prejudice. As late as the 1960s, the male-dominated medical profession and the various ruling bodies in athletics believed it was dangerous for women to take part in the marathon. It was left to women themselves to change these attitudes. In 1964 the Scottish runner, Dale Grieg, was the first woman to break the three hour 30 minutes barrier, but the authorities sent an ambulance to follow her all the way to the finish line! Three years later, Kathrine Switzer entered the Boston Marathon without indicating her sex. She was assumed to be male and turned up at the start-line wearing a hood. Seconds before the start she discarded the hood, revealing her gender. Realising their mistake, the race director and several officials ran after her but were unable to catch her!

I can still remember with some embarrassment the time I foolishly joined a keep-fit class run by the local ladies hockey team. All went well for the first 20 minutes as I mockingly exaggerated the movements of the exercises. We then moved on to stretching, and I was still enjoying the music and the attention I was getting from the class, when I was gripped by the worst bout of cramp I have ever experienced. I limped away, complaining of an old rugby injury, amid a fanfare of giggles. Mentally, women are very strong and highly motivated; however, prejudice aside, they are faced with certain anatomical and physiological differences which prevent them from achieving the same power-output as men.

These include:

- A small heart volume, with cardiac output around 10 per cent lower than an equivalent male.
- Approximately a 20 per cent reduction in blood volume for the same body weight.
- Less of the oxygen carrying blood protein and a 10 per cent reduction in vital capacity.
- A wider pelvis which increases the angle of the thigh bone and brings the knees closer together.
- Around 10 per cent more body fat than a man of the same body weight.
- A shorter Achilles tendon resulting in a diminished elastic recoil when running.
- A menstrual cycle which imposes its own pressures on a woman's body and mind, and may diminish overall performance.

This list of differences is put into perspective when we consider that women have won gold medals in all sports and, incidentally, during all of the different phases of their menstrual cycle. In fact, regular exercise and fitness training offer some distinct advantages for women:

- Exercise and fitness training have been shown to decrease menstrual pain.
- Pre-menstrual tension (PMT) can be reduced by regular exercise.
- Swimming, cycling and aerobic walking are particularly well-suited to pregnancy, and all exercise raises blood oxygen which is very beneficial for the foetus.
- Exercise can relieve pregnancy-associated problems such as excessive weight gain, constipation, morning sickness and varicose veins.
- Reduction in the length of labour by some $2^1/_2$ hours in the first phase and 20 minutes in the second phase has been observed in some athletes.
- Exercise is 'anti-depressive' and elevates mood during pregnancy.

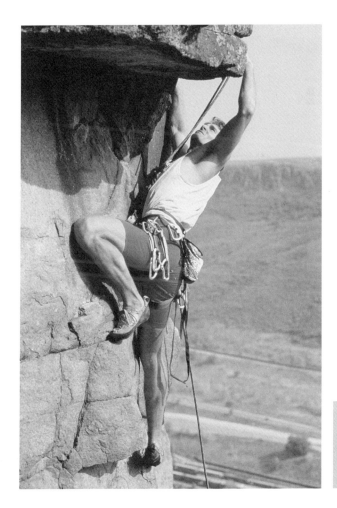

Building strength,
stamina and overall
fitness can lead you to
take up challenging
outdoor pursuits,
such as rock climbing,
which revitalise both
body and spirit.

However, regular exercise can disrupt the menstrual cycle and menstruation can cease altogether. This is a response to stress and a normal cycle should resume as soon as training is stopped or reduced. If you are worried, speak to your doctor.

Many women continue to exercise during pregnancy but this should be discussed with your doctor. As a general rule, new fitness programmes should never be initiated during pregnancy. Swimming, cycling and walking are better than running. A pregnant woman should never race or run for long periods, since a decreased blood flow to the womb can damage the unborn baby. Equally, she should not allow herself to become overheated, since an elevated body temperature can damage the foetus.

It is important for women to dress correctly when exercising. The breast has no muscles for support; instead, it depends on fibrous tissues which stretch during exercise. Therefore, a fully supportive sports bra is strongly recommended.

Selecting a Gym

It is important to select the right gym or fitness centre. It often pays to visit a number in the area before making your selection. The nearest centre may not be the best one! Here are a few points to help you make the right decision.

- The gym should provide instructors with nationally recognised qualifications. A good instructor should demonstrate the exercises, offer support and be constructively critical of your performance, while showing you ways of improving.
- There should be a pleasant, friendly atmosphere.
- Lockers should be available to hold clothing and valuables.
- The club should have good changing and showering facilities and should be spotlessly clean.
- Floor space is very important for warm-ups and training. There should be at least one area which allows you sufficient freedom of movement.
- A jaccuzi, sauna or steam room is a nice place to relax after exercise – but do not overdo it!
- The gym should be well-equipped with exercise machines and free weights. Members of staff should be on hand to organise training and prevent individuals from hogging the machines.

There are other alternatives to health clubs and fitness centres. The YMCA often has excellent facilities and at a fraction of the price of more commercial outlets. Schools and colleges usually offer spacious gyms and some offer training sessions in the evening. Of course, you can always train at home, but lack of space may be a problem. On fine days, you can always use the garden. Self-motivation may be another problem; there are no gym instructors to spur you on! You will have to buy your own sports equipment but this need not be too difficult or expensive. You can rig up some simple exercise machines such as punch bags and speed balls in the garage. Buy a skipping rope. A bench is advisable, ideally with leg extensions and a dip bar. Invest in good quality iron weights. You will need a set of weights that can be secured on a bar or dumb-bell. The set should increase in 1 kg (2½lb) increments and consist of 1, 5, 10 15, 20 kg (2½, 12, 25, 35 and 45 lb) plates. The weights need good collars that can be changed quickly. Never lift or use weights which are not secured – they can cause serious injuries.

The SAS Warm-Up

Any moderate exercise, such as jogging, is an ideal warm-up but all the muscle groups need to be worked. Walking, swimming and cycling can all be used as long as you take it steady. The general idea is to raise the pulse and get the blood circulating. The length of time spent warming up will depend on the ambient temperature. On a warm day, the minimum warm-up period is about six minutes, but on a cold day you will need to exercise for approximately 12 minutes.

Warming Up in a Gym

- Jog around the gym. For the first three laps stay on your toes and exaggerate the knee lift.
- Start to exercise the arms on the fourth lap. Punch the arms high, first with the left arm and then with the right.
- On lap five, face inwards and run sideways, leading with the left leg. Half-way through the lap, face outwards so that your right leg leads.
- On the next lap (lap six), hop for 10 m (33 ft) on one leg then change to the other.
- On lap seven, run backwards for half a lap and then forward again, punching your arms above your head. When the seven laps are

complete, stand with your legs one shoulder's width apart, with hands on hips and elbows slightly forward. Breathe deeply, inhaling through the nose and out through the mouth.

Shuttle Runs

Select three lines about 10 m (33 ft) apart. You can use white lines on the gym floor, or they can be imaginary, or perhaps marked out with small objects such as coins. Just how long you make each line depends on your overall fitness. It is better to start with short lines of approximately 10–20 m (33–66 ft) in length.

Sprint to the end of the first line, touch the floor with the palm of your hand and sprint back to the start. Repeat the exercise for the middle and furthest line and return to the start. This is one set or repetition. Repeat this twice more to complete three sets. These shuttle runs are killers and really separate the men from the boys.

Using the same lines, we repeat the exercise, only this time we do five press-ups before sprinting back to the start. Run to the end of the middle line and do five 'burpees' (see page 30 for instructions) before sprinting back. Now run to furthest line and do five 'crunches' (see pages 32–33 for instructions) and return.

Repeat three times with a 30-second rest period between each set. Recover from the exercise with deep breathing until your respiration rate and heart rate have returned to normal.

REMEMBER: This warm-up period helps to prevent injury and prepares us for hard exercise. It should never be omitted.

Warming Up in a Restricted Space

Gyms are often crowded with either people or apparatus and it may not be possible to perform the sort of exercises described above. In this case, alternative warm-up routines will have to be found. You could run or cycle to the gym or perhaps the gym has exercise machines such as treadmills. Cycling machines and treadmills offer some very distinct advantages. Speed and distance can be varied on treadmills, while some tilt, simulating running uphill. The machines, being indoors, are not 'weather dependent'. You are also mercifully saved from dogs, traffic and chilly winds. The machines exercise the cardio-vascular system and tone the muscles under the watchful eye of the gym instructor. Rowing machines are another variation on this theme. Some of these allow you to race against a rival crew. The graphics are great and at the very least you will not be bored! At the end of the warm-up, you are not far from a hot cup of something and a warm shower.

Warming Up Outdoors

You may be far from a gym but you can always warm up outdoors. The great difference is that if the weather is cold, a longer time must be spent on the warm-up and care must be taken if you are to avoid damaging cold muscles.

To warm up outdoors, you need to find an area of at least 25 x 25 m (82 x 82 ft). This should be large enough to complete the circuit and shuttle runs described on page 15. The great advantage of outdoor training is that the space and fresh air are free! But take care to check that the ground you are to use is free from holes or humps that could cause you to turn and damage your ankles or trip you up.

Flexing and Stretching

When stretching we should always start at the top and work down.

Head and Neck

- Stand easily with hands on hips and legs one shoulder's width apart. Rotate your head in a large circle, taking care to flex back as far as is comfortable and brush the upper chest with the chin. Do six repetitions clockwise and six counter-clockwise.
- Now turn the head left and right, trying to see as far behind you as possible. Try to work up to 12 repetitions. Do this slowly at first.

As your exercise programme progresses, the neck muscles will become more flexible and you will be able to do this at a faster rate.

- Bend the head forwards until the chin touches the chest. Gradually flex the head back until you are looking at the sky. Repeat the exercise, starting to move your head to the right. Do six 'nods' to the left and six to the right.

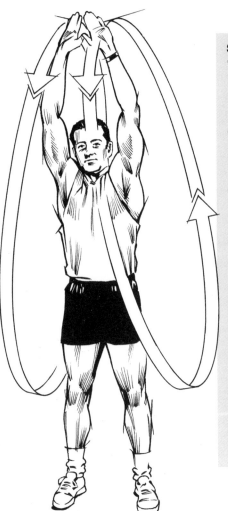

Shoulders

- Stand as usual with your legs one shoulder's width apart. Hold your arms parallel to the ground, fists slightly clenched. Circle the arms forwards for 12 repetitions and again backwards for 12 repetitions.
- To practice co-ordination, do another 12 repetitions, only this time move the arms in opposite directions. Practice changing the direction of rotation of both arms.
- We now continue the exercise while bending forward at the waist until the upper body is parallel to the ground. Do three repetitions on the way down and three on the way back up. Rotating your arms while bending forward is easy but revolving your arms while returning to the upright position requires more practice. This helps to perfect co-ordination.
- Next, we start the exercise with the arms extended at the shoulder. Raise your arms above your head until the palms touch and then slap them down on the outside of the knees. Do 12 repetitions.
- Stand up straight and circle your arms, keeping them as close to the body as possible. Do 12 repetitions forwards and another 12 in the reverse direction.

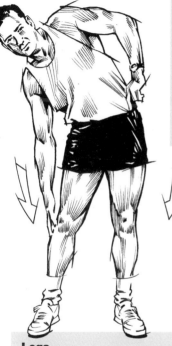

Trunk

- Stand with left hand on hip, legs shoulder width apart. Bend to the right forcing the right hand to slide down to touch the right ankle. Remember, do not bend at the knees or allow the body to lean forwards. Repeat the exercise bending to the left. Do 12 repetitions on each side.
- Standing with legs apart, try and place the palms of the hand on the ground as you reach forwards, back, left, right and then centre. Return to the standing position slowly. Do 12 repetitions in total.

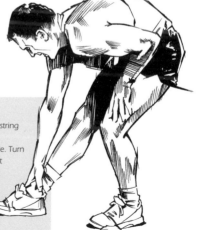

Legs

We finally finish our warm up by stretching the hamstring muscles in the leg.

- Stand upright with legs as wide apart as possible. Turn and pivot to the right, bending the left knee but keeping the right leg straight. Reach down and hold the right ankle for three seconds. Do six repetitions on each leg.
- To end the warm-up, jog three slow laps of the gym, shaking out the limbs.

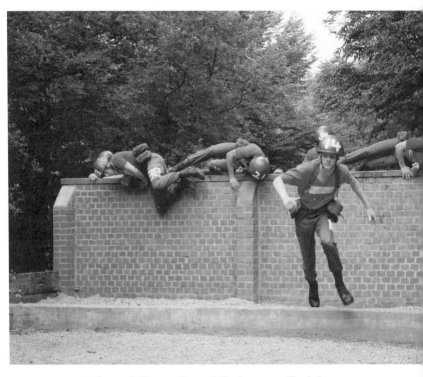

An SAS-style assault course offers one of the best opportunities for speed, strength and endurance training. Devise your own course (see page 43).

Speed, Strength and Endurance Training

There are a wide range of exercises we can do to build up our strength, speed and stamina, falling under such headings as:

Callisthenics: These are the rigid, military-type, 'parade ground' exercises, designed to promote straight backs, raised chests and a shoulders-back attitude. Some regard a rigid military bearing as a painfully unnatural position but there are others willing to take a pride in themselves and undergo slight discomfort to look and feel the part. As the old adage goes 'If you look good, you feel good'.

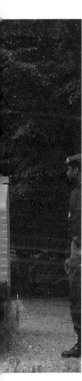

Anaerobic Exercise: Very few exercises are anaerobic. Anaerobic exercises tend to be fast, furious and short. During this type of exercise, energy and power are generated in the muscles without using oxygen from the blood. So this sort of exercise does not depend on regulating your breathing or having muscles well supplied with blood vessels. It is also very inefficient, producing only 10 per cent of the available energy compared to aerobic processes. Of all the standard track events, only the 100 metres is run without using oxygen from the blood. The essence of the 100 metres is, of course, fast sprinting, and this has led some doctors to speculate that anaerobic respiration was developed to provide early man with a short, fast burst of speed which helped him out-run predators.

Aerobic Exercise: Most exercise is aerobic, requiring increased heart and lung capacity. Aerobic exercise also includes endurance work-outs such as rowing, cycling and swimming and the longer track events such as the 800 and 1500 metres and, of course, the marathon. Aerobic exercise helps develop heart and lung capacity vital to overall fitness.

Interval Training: Interval training is an extensive work-out which builds up speed and strength without using weights. Intensive periods of exercise interspersed with short rest periods enable you to work longer and more efficiently. During each short 'recovery' period, the chemicals responsible for fatigue, such as lactic acid, are cleared from the muscles, energy-rich chemicals are regenerated and blood oxygen saturates the tissues.

Circuit Training: Circuit training is similar to interval training but here we include weights and exercise machines. You should aim to exercise all of the muscle groups in the body and complete as many repetitions in a given time as possible, before moving on to the next exercise.

Weight Training: This increases performance by increasing our strength. It also develops muscles which protect vulnerable areas, such as the straight muscles of the abdomen that guard the solar plexus against blows.

CHAPTER TWO

Strength Training Without Weights

This first part of our training programme involves exercises which need no special equipment and can be done anywhere. Sometimes the SAS soldier finds himself in a remote area with limited resources or perhaps within the confines of hotel room. He uses this programme to keep fit. I recommend that novices start here. This regime will exercise all the body and prepare you for more arduous programmes later in the book.

WARNING: Do you suffer from any of the following conditions?
- High blood pressure
- Heart disorders
- Respiratory problems
- Blood disorders
- Muscle and bone problems
- Obesity

If the answer is yes, seek medical advice before attempting any exercise programme. The same advice should be followed by those over 40 years of age, pregnant women and those with a specific health problem.

We are going to split the exercises in this section into three types: aerobic, anaerobic and exercises to work the abdominal muscles. Obviously, maximum benefit is obtained by mixing these types of exercise in any one session. We always warm up and then we alternate between anaerobic/aerobic exercises and exercises to work the abdominal muscles. I cannot stress the importance of building strong abdominal muscles. Much of our strength, speed and power comes from these muscle groups and all too often they are overlooked. Become familiar with these basic exercises. Follow the instructions carefully and try to do them properly.

REMEMBER: if you cheat you are only cheating yourself.

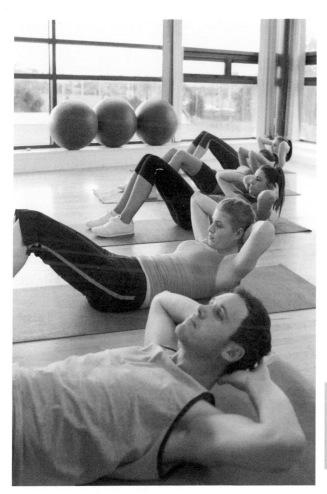

The exercises presented in this chapter require no specialist equipment and very little space. However, working out in a group or class is both motivating and highly enjoyable.

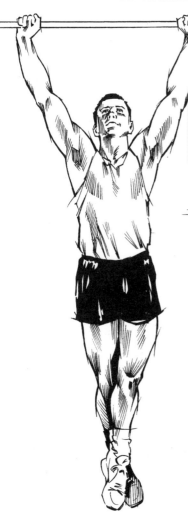

Chins

An excellent exercise for the upper body and triceps.

- Reach up and take a wide overhand grip on a bar situated high enough to just let your legs dangle off the floor.
- Cross your legs and pull yourself up until your chin bone brushes the bar.
- Lower until your arms are fully extended.

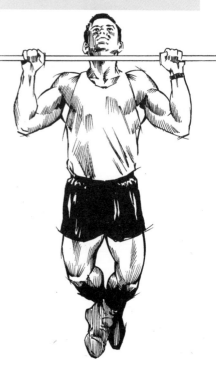

Lunges

A good work-out of the thighs and upper leg muscles.

- Place the hands behind the neck and move one leg forward, taking a longer stride than usual.
- Bend the leading leg until the thigh is parallel with the ground.
- Repeat the exercise using the other leg.

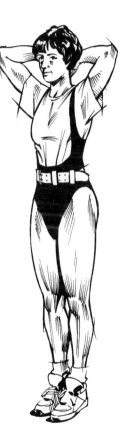

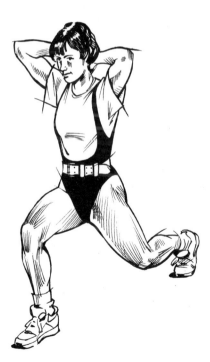

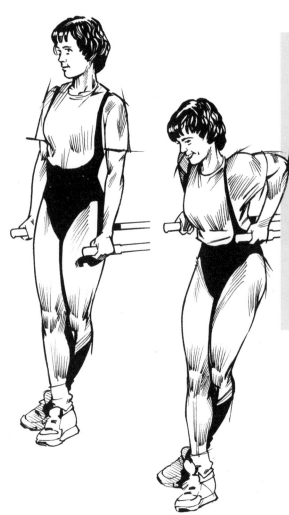

Parallel Dips

- You will need two parallel bars raised about 1.2 m (4 ft) off the ground and placed approximately one shoulder width apart (you can improvise with furniture).
- Grip both bars, cross your legs and raise your body off the ground by locking your arms.
- Now lower your body until your elbows are level with the bars, keeping your feet clear of the floor.
- Finally, return to the start position.

A difficult exercise initially, but well worth the effort to produce good results.

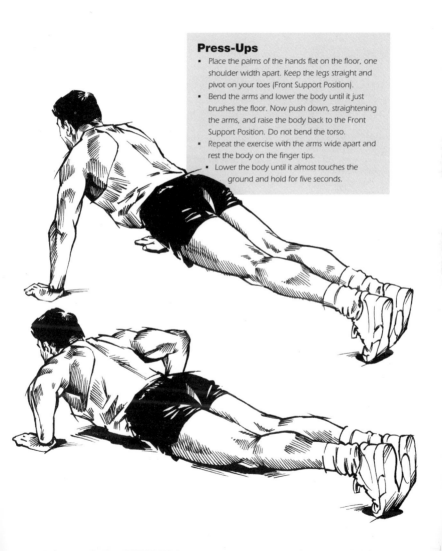

Press-Ups

- Place the palms of the hands flat on the floor, one shoulder width apart. Keep the legs straight and pivot on your toes (Front Support Position).
- Bend the arms and lower the body until it just brushes the floor. Now push down, straightening the arms, and raise the body back to the Front Support Position. Do not bend the torso.
- Repeat the exercise with the arms wide apart and rest the body on the finger tips.
- Lower the body until it almost touches the ground and hold for five seconds.

Calf Raises

- Stand on a platform approximately 10cm (4 in) high (two stacked telephone directories would be ideal).
- Raise yourself onto the balls of your feet.
- Raise one leg behind you, maintaining balance by holding onto a wall.
- Raise the body onto the toes before sinking down below the level of the platform.

This really tones the calf muscles! Repeat the exercise using the other leg.

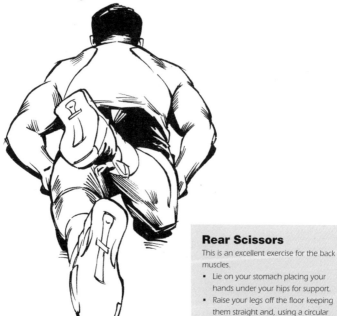

Rear Scissors

This is an excellent exercise for the back muscles.

- Lie on your stomach placing your hands under your hips for support.
- Raise your legs off the floor keeping them straight and, using a circular motion, cross the right leg over the left leg.

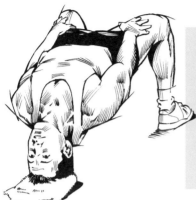

Reverse Neck Roll

This exercise builds a strong neck which is essential for the martial arts. You might experience stiffness initially but do not give up on this vital exercise.

- With your head on the ground, make a Wrestler's Bridge with your hands on your thighs. Protect the top of your head with something soft (a broad cushion is ideal for this).
- Now lean forward until your full body weight is taken by your head and neck.

Head Roll

- Kneel with knees slightly apart and then lean forward to place your forehead on the ground in front of you.
- Place your hands on the back of your thighs and gradually roll forward until your body weight is placed onto your neck. Use a rolling motion to increase the pressure.

TAKE CARE WITH THIS EXERCISE! DO IT GENTLY AT FIRST AND MAKE SURE THAT YOUR BODY IS WELL BALANCED.

CAUTION: The two neck exercises above should only be done under strict supervision. They are very demanding and should only be attempted if you have no history of neck or back problems. Build up slowly!

Alternative Neck Exercises

- Try to do the full range of neck movements wearing a close fitting harness with weights attached.
- Stand up and bend forward for one set, raising and lowering your neck.
- Lie on a bench face up with your shoulders supporting your neck and head. Raise and lower your head slowly.

Aerobic Exercises

Squat Thrusts

- From the Front Support Position (see Press-Ups, page 27), snap your legs forward until your knees touch your elbows, then shoot both legs back to the Front Support Position.

A good exercise for the arms and legs, it gets the old pulse racing!

Burpees

- Starting again from the Front Support Position, bring your knees up to your elbows, but this time leap up as high as possible, before returning to the squat position and then shooting your legs backwards.

Stride Jumps

- Stand astride a box about 46 cm (18 in) high (a stool is ideal).
- Jump up lightly bringing both feet together above the box and return to the astride position.

Alternative Stride Jumping

- Using the same box or stool, jump up and down twice and on the third repetition jump clear of the box.
- Land, keeping feet and knees together and repeat.

Step-Ups

- Use two boxes - one 46 cm (18 in) high and the other 91 cm (36 in) high. Step onto the lower box with the left leg and the top box with the right leg and then move the left leg alongside. You should now have both feet on the top box.
- Now, step back onto the lower box and finally back onto the floor. If you do not have good, sturdy boxes, the stairs will do nicely. Do as many repetitions as you can. Practise alternating the leading leg; this is good for improving your co-ordination.

Jump-Ups

- Stand with feet together in front of the 46-cm 18-in) box. Jump onto the box, landing with feet and knees together, using your arms to propel you.

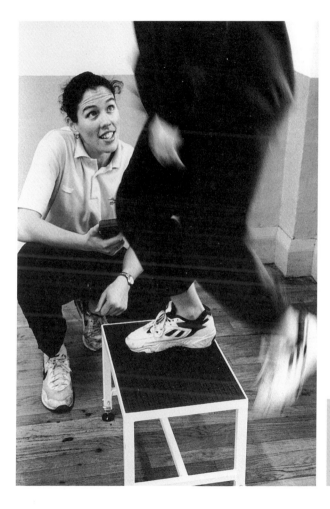

As a variation, step up onto the box with your right leg and stand on top. Then step down, starting with the left leg. Repeat with your left leg. Continue to alternate legs.

Abdominal Exercises

The great exterior muscles of the abdomen, thorax and back, which are of interest to the keep-fit enthusiast, sportsman and martial artist, fall into several well-known groups. These muscles are attached to bone by white, fibrous, inelastic cords called tendons. Other structures called ligaments attach bone to bone or serve to support the internal organs. The greater pectoral muscles cover both sides of the chest running from either side of the breast-bone to the armpit. Below the pectorals, the external oblique muscle of the abdomen runs from the groin to cover the sides of the body, interweaving with anterior serratus muscles above the rib-cage. The internal and external oblique muscles help to rotate and flex the trunk. All of these muscles intermesh with the straight muscle of the abdomen which runs from the chest to the groin (noticeably flaccid in middle-aged spread and brewer's belly but nicely rippled in body builders).

On the back, the great trapezius muscles cover the neck and ribs running from the midline of the body to the shoulders. These partly cover the two latissimus dorsi which run from the lower spine, across the ribs, to cover the sides of the body. Behind the shoulders, and in a triangle between the trapezius and the latissimus dorsi, are found the infraspinous muscles and the teres minor and teres major.

Thigh Hand Slide

- Lie on your back.
- Press your chin against your chest and place your hands on top of your thighs.
- Now, slide your hands down along your thighs until you reach your knees, slowly raising your upper body clear of the ground by a least 10 cm (4 in).
- Recover and then repeat the exercise.

The 'V' Crunch

- Lie once again on your back with your legs raised some 45 degrees off the ground.
- With your hands inter-locked behind your neck, sit up and touch your knees with your forehead.

A difficult exercise but an excellent one to check the progress of your abdominal muscles. Do not allow yourself to be defeated!

Crunches

- Lie on your back with your hands behind your head.
- Bring both knees up together, at the same time raising your head to meet them over the torso. Keep your knees raised and stationary for as long as possible.
- Finally, lower head and knees back to the floor.

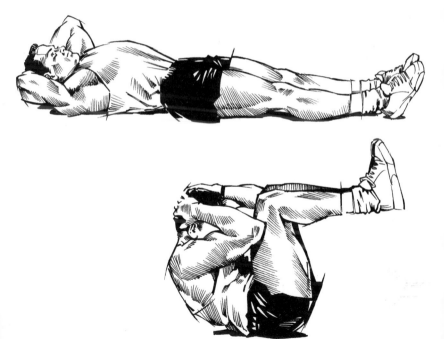

Sit-Ups

- Place your feet under a bar (or a piece of furniture) or perhaps you can persuade a companion to hold them.
- Place your hands behind your head and, keeping legs straight, sit up.
- Lower your body back to the floor.

You will feel the tension in the abdominal muscles as they work to raise your body!

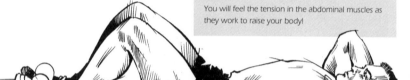

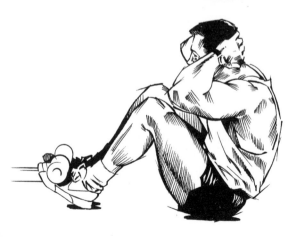

Twisting Crunches

- Lie on the floor with your hands behind your head.
- This time, as you raise your legs and upper body, twist your torso so that your left elbow touches your right knee.
- Repeat, alternating left and right elbows to touch right and left knees. Feel that stretch at your waist!

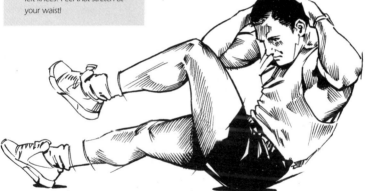

Bent Knee Sit-Ups

- Again, lie on your back, with knees bent, feet on the ground and hands behind your neck.
- Sit up, touching your chin to your knees.
- Now finish the exercise by lowering your upper body until it is parallel with, but not touching, the floor.

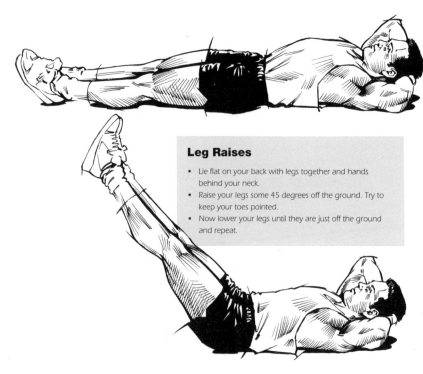

Leg Raises

- Lie flat on your back with legs together and hands behind your neck.
- Raise your legs some 45 degrees off the ground. Try to keep your toes pointed.
- Now lower your legs until they are just off the ground and repeat.

Straight Leg Raises

- Lie flat with legs extended and place your hands, palms down, under your buttocks.
- Keeping your legs straight and, pointing your toes, raise your legs until they are just beyond the vertical.
- Lower and repeat the exercise but keep your feet off the ground between repetitions.

This exercise puts a lot of strain on the lower back but is one of the best work-outs for the straight muscle of the abdomen.

Programme One

Before we start, we must always remember to warm up and stretch those muscles. Remember, flexibility is very important. A loose body goes with a relaxed mind. Do not make the common mistake of eating prior to exercise. Personally, I prefer to get up early in the morning to do a work-out and then shower and eat breakfast.

Wear a T-shirt under a sweat vest, with shorts and jockey pants, swimming trunks or a jock-strap to support the genitals. A supportive bra is essential for women following this programme. Wear a tracksuit over the training gear. This can be removed when you warm up.

WARM-UP	6 MINUTES
STRETCHING	2 MINUTES

EXERCISE	REPETITIONS	SETS
PRESS-UPS	5	3
CRUNCHES	5	3
LUNGES	5	3
LEG RAISES	5	3
DIPS	5	3
BENT KNEE SIT-UPS	5	3
CALF RAISES	5	3
THIGH HAND SLIDES	5	3
CHINS	5	3
LEG RAISES	5	3
REAR SCISSORS	5	3
SIT-UPS	5	3

Work as hard as possible and move straight on to the next exercise. Each set should take no more than two minutes to perform. After the first set, take a three-minute rest.

Do not progress on to the other programmes in this manual until you can do each set of exercises in under two minutes.

Warm-Down

Just as it is very important to warm up before exercise, it is also important to 'warm down' after hard exercise. This ensures that the pulse rate and other body functions can gradually return to normal. During hard exercise, the circular bands of smooth muscle surrounding some veins are squeezed to help return blood to the heart. Another feature of the 'venous return' mechanism is the system of valves in larger veins which impedes backflow. During warming down, this venous return mechanism is kept operating to prevent dizziness and fainting. We really only appreciate this back-up system when it fails – for example when a soldier faints on parade. Another reason for warming down is that it ensures that the build-up of lactic acid is cleared from the muscles more efficiently. Warming down is very important in pregnancy and for women who have recently given birth, since changes in the body during pregnancy leave joints very susceptible to injury. These changes result from the release of relaxin, a hormone which loosens joints and connective tissue, particularly in the pelvis, in preparation for birth. These changes persist for some weeks after delivery.

Jog around the gym, shaking out the arms, shoulders and neck. Then stand, feet apart, and cycle the arms backwards and forwards for 10 repetitions in each direction. Stand with your feet apart and try to touch the floor in front, now stretching to touch the ground to the left and right. Repeat this last exercise for 10 repetitions and then breathe deeply in through the nose and out through the mouth, until your breathing returns to normal. Now, as part of the warm-down, here are some stretching exercises to try.

Hamstring Stretch

- Stand with your feet together and legs straight.
- Bending forward at the waist and keeping your back straight, reach down in one smooth motion and grasp your ankles.
- Stretch a little more, applying gentle pressure on the hamstrings.
- Return to the upright position.
- Do this to a count of four. Count to four as you bend forward, hold for four and count to four as you return to the upright position. Try 10 repetitions of this exercise.

Seated Hamstring Stretch

- Sit on the floor, legs straight out in front.
- Bend forward and grasp your ankles, gently pulling forward to stretch the hamstrings.

Do this exercise to a count of four and perform 10 repetitions.

Legs-Apart Hamstring Stretch

- Sit on the floor with your legs as wide apart as possible.
- Keep your back straight and reach forward to grasp your left ankle.
- Hold for a count of four and then change to grasp the right ankle.

Seated Side Bend

- Remain on the floor, legs spread as wide as possible.
- Raise your right arm over your head and lean as far to the left as possible.
- Now try and touch your left ankle.
- Hold the ankle for a count of four and repeat the exercise on the other side. Do 10 repetitions of each.

Back Stretch

◆ Sit on a table, close to an edge, with your companion holding your ankles and lean back so that your body clears the table and your head is lowered to the floor. Do 10 repetitions.

Walk around the gym for three laps, while silently assessing your performance. What were your strengths and weaknesses? If you find that you are cooling down too quickly, put on your sweat vest and track suit.

You might have a few aches and pains but you can console yourself with these thoughts. As your heart and circulatory system become more efficient, the risks of heart disease and hypertension diminish. During exercise more blood flows through the muscles and internal organs, increasing their efficiency. Prolonged exercise builds muscle and burns calories. Your body and stamina will improve and you will feel more energetic and confident.

Programme Two

When you have mastered the first programme and can complete it in the times allowed, it is time to progress. Put as much effort into these exercises as possible, with only three minutes rest between each set.

WARM-UP	6 MINUTES
STRETCHING	2 MINUTES

EXERCISE	REPETITIONS	SETS
SQUAT THRUSTS	5	3
CRUNCHES	5	3
BURPEES	5	3
STRIDE JUMPS	5	3
BENT KNEE SIT-UPS	5	3
ALTERNATE STRIDES	5	3
THIGH HAND SLIDES	5	3
STEP-UPS	5	3
LEG RAISES	5	3
JUMP-UPS	5	3
SIT-UPS	5	3

Quadriceps Stretch

- Stand with your right hand against a wall for support (or grasp the back of a chair).
- Reach down and grasp your left foot at the instep and draw the heel towards the buttocks.
- Hold for 30 seconds.
- Slowly let go of your foot and repeat the exercise with your right leg.

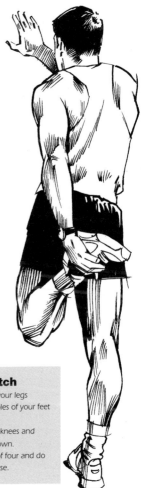

Inner Thigh Stretch

- Remain seated and draw your legs towards you so that the soles of your feet touch.
- Place your hands on your knees and gently force your knees down.
- Again, do this to a count of four and do 10 repetitions of the exercise.

Programme Three

This programme incorporates the previous two work-outs. This routine
will take a lot of effort and some time to achieve. It alternates between
anaerobic, aerobic and abdominal exercises and should be completed in
less than six minutes.

WARM-UP	6 MINUTES	
STRETCHING	2 MINUTES	

EXERCISE	REPETITIONS	SETS
PRESS-UPS	10	3
CRUNCHES	10	3
SQUAT THRUSTS	10	3
STRAIGHT LEG RAISES	10	3
DIPS	10	3
BENT KNEE SIT-UPS	10	3
BURPEES	10	3
THIGH HAND SLIDES	10	3
CHINS	10	3
LEG RAISES	10	3
STRIDE JUMPS	10	3
SIT-UPS	10	3
CALF RAISES	10	3
CRUNCHIES	10	3
STEP-UPS	10	3
STRAIGHT LEG RAISES	10	3
LUNGES	10	3
BENT KNEE SIT-UPS	10	3
JUMP-UPS	10	3
THIGH HAND SLIDES	10	3
REAR SCISSORS	10	3
LEG RAISES	10	3

Additional Routine

Once you have completed Programme Three in the minimum target time of six minutes, add the following exercises to the basic regime for an even greater challenge!

WARM-UP	6 MINUTES
STRETCHING	2 MINUTES

EXERCISE	REPETITIONS	SETS
HEAD ROLLS	10	3
TWISTING CRUNCHES	10	3
PARALLEL DIPS	10	3
'V' CRUNCHES	10	3
REVERSE NECK ROLLS	10	3
ROPE CLIMB	10	3
CHINS	10 OVERHAND	
CHINS	10 UNDERHAND	

The SAS Assault Course

One of the finest overall fitness routines is the assault course. It demands constant changes of pace and exercises all the major muscle groups. It is excellent for the heart and lungs, building strength, speed, stamina and co-ordination.

You can build your own assault course on open ground or in a gym. The idea is to make a series of obstacles that constantly challenge you, like going under bars, climbing ropes and vaulting obstacles.

On an outdoor course you can make use of natural features such as the sides of hills, streams, gullies, trenches and so on. You should build obstacles that force you to jump over them or climb underneath them.

When faced with building an assault course indoors, you have to be imaginative. Put a bench on two chairs to crawl under or go over. Try rigging up a rope to climb. Bring out the parallel bars and negotiate these. Mark out two lines, 2 m (6½ ft) apart, and pretend that it is a bottomless chasm.

CHAPTER THREE

Strength Training With Weights

The exercises in the previous chapter will get you super fit and will start to develop body strength. To progress, we must introduce weight training. Training for strength involves short, intensive periods of work interspersed with longer periods of rest. There are no short-cuts. Increasing the workload too quickly only results in bunched, strained and torn muscles. Tendons which connect muscles to bone can become inflamed and even damaged. No matter how far you run or swim, or how hard you exercise, you always contract your muscles against the same amount of resistance. As you improve and run longer distances or exercise for longer periods, you will build up your endurance but you will not become any stronger. A strong, muscular body gives protection to the vital organs inside the body and is more resistant to injury. Specific weight-training regimes can help you with your chosen sport.

Some people believe that weight training will make you sluggish and inflexible. This can be true but only if the training is done incorrectly. By following the exercises in *The SAS Personal Trainer*, you will gain added mobility, especially if you are in the over-40 age group. Incorporated with the other fitness programmes in this manual, weight training will help you to develop greater speed, power and endurance. The great advantage of weight training is that you can actually see the progress you are making.

Muscles

Muscles are the meat on the frame of the body, accounting for nearly half of its weight. Those that are of interest to us are the skeletal muscles. They come in various sizes and shapes and are connected in different ways to the bones. Muscle groups involved in the movement or rotation of the body work in opposition to each other (they are said to be 'antagonistic'), so that when one group is contracted, the other group is relaxed.

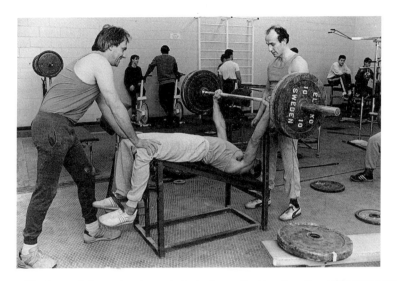

Muscles work by contracting and shortening, pulling together the bones which are attached to the ends of the muscles. Normal contractions are termed 'concentric'. For example, you can see the biceps in the arm bulging when a weight is lifted.

Isometric or 'static' contractions occur when the force of the contraction exactly equals, or is less than, the force preventing movement. We see this when a weight is held at arm's length or when you try to push against a wall. Let us take the example of the wall. The wall does not move but neither do your arm muscles, despite a very great effort and expenditure of energy. The forces developed within the muscles are, in fact, greatest for these isometric contractions; muscles work most efficiently when their change in length is small. However, as the muscles are working hard without contracting (and allowing the release of lactic acid), they become fatigued very quickly.

Some contractions are termed 'eccentric', when the force exerted on the muscle is greater than the force of contraction. We see these

Training partners can prove invaluable in providing motivation, camaraderie and practical assistance in doing certain exercises and helping with over-heavy weights.

contractions when a weight-lifter releases a very heavy weight, or in the leg (quadriceps) muscles of someone running downhill. Not surprisingly, muscle and tendon damage occurs more frequently during eccentric contractions than during normal concentric contractions.

Muscles are composed of many fibres which vary in length from 1-60 mm ($1/20$-$2\frac{1}{2}$ in) and in thickness from around 10 to 100 micrometers (that is from a $1/5$-$1/15$ of the diameter of a strand of human hair). These fibres are actually the cells which shorten when the muscle contracts. The composition of fibres in muscle varies, not only from muscle to muscle but from individual to individual. This is why some of us are good at endurance sports, while others perform better as sprinters. In animals, the situation is often very clear cut. In some fish, so-called white muscle predominates which is poorly supplied with blood vessels, and energy generation is therefore primarily anaerobic. These animals are fitted to be 'sprinters', either racing to escape predators or to catch their own prey. As most anglers are aware, the hooked fish fights hard at first but very soon tires. In contrast, the flight muscles of migratory birds are packed with blood vessels (so-called red muscle) and generate their energy aerobically. Red muscle is designed for endurance. The situation in human muscle is more complex, since all muscles contain both red and white fibres.

There are at least three different fibres; slow-twitch, fast-twitch glycolytic and fast-twitch oxidative, and they differ as to how they generate the necessary energy to contract.

Slow-Twitch Oxidative: Aerobic fibres most abundant in red muscle. They contract slowly and are relatively fatigue resistant.

Fast-Twitch Glycolytic: These fibres generate their energy anaerobically. They are most common in white muscle and are easily fatigued.

Fast-Twitch Oxidative: These fibres use both anaerobic and aerobic processes. They contract rapidly and are intermediate in their susceptibility to fatigue.

Just as the different muscles in the body will differ in the various proportions of these three fibres, so the proportions will vary between individuals. While training plays a role in developing the types of muscle an athlete needs for his or her sport, our genetic heritage supplies the controlling influence; some of us are natural sprinters and some are endurance sportsmen and women. A person with predominately slow-

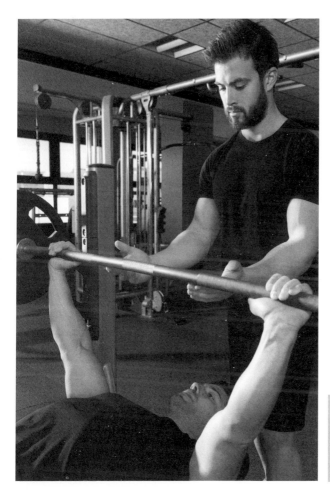

In weight training, always aim for a fluid, controlled movement; never jerk up a weight. Concentrate your mind on the muscles you are working, in this case the biceps.

twitch oxidative fibres in his or her leg muscles has the necessary 'equipment' to excel at the marathon but will never reach the speeds of the top-class sprinter.

Muscles are frequently grouped in the body. For example, the quadriceps of the thigh are composed of four muscles: the vastus medialis, rectus femoris, vastus intermedialis and the vastus lateralis. These latin names are rather formidable and some time ago, the decision was taken to replace these with more descriptive names. Hence the quadriceps group was renamed the straight muscle of the thigh, the lateral great muscle, intermediate dorsal muscle and medial inferior muscle. I mention this as nomenclature varies from book to book and it can become rather confusing.

The important muscle groups in limbs are frequently arranged in antagonistic pairs working against each other. One such pair are the quadriceps and biceps muscles of the thigh. The biceps contract to raise the thigh during walking, by flexing the knee joint. The quadriceps remain relaxed. As the foot is placed back on the ground, the quadriceps extend the leg and the biceps of the thigh relax.

Other muscles work to control and stabilise the joint during flexion of the limb. This is important when joints can move in several directions, allowing both flexion and rotation. Muscles can also work to prevent the over-extension of a joint, thus protecting the joint capsule and vulnerable soft tissue.

How Often to Train

It is best to use weights every second day, having a day's rest period in- between. During a work-out with weights, the muscle fibres are developed by working them against a high degree of resistance. After such a work-out, it is important to give those muscles time to recover.

How Much Weight?

Starting with light weights and doing the full range of movements enables us to strengthen muscle groups without losing speed and agility. By doing multiple repetitions, we develop the muscles, thus gaining strength and power. If we only work with heavy weights, we will increase muscle bulk and power but this will be at the expense of speed and agility.

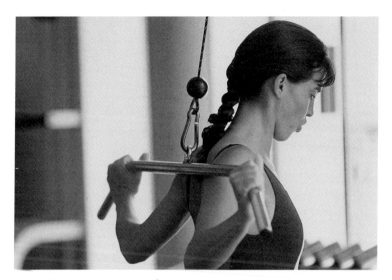

Duration of Training Period

The minimum period of weight training, with warming-up and cooling-down periods, is around 45 minutes. The best approach is to take it steady until you are familiar and comfortable with the routine and can exercise all the muscle groups. Towards the end of each session, you can concentrate on one particular muscle group and give the muscles a good work-out. To prevent your training programme from becoming too boring, we can split the session to work:

1 Shoulders and chest
2 Arms and back
3 Legs

Although free weights are the most effective tools in weight training, certain weight machines offer useful additional exercises, including this pull-down bar.

You may soon notice that blisters and calluses start to develop on the palms of your hands from handling the weights. If the discomfort becomes too great, you can always buy a pair of weight-lifter's gloves. These have no fingers and strong, padded palms. The back is another area vulnerable to injury. It can be protected and supported by a wide leather belt. The belt is worn for power exercises and removed for abdominal and floor work.

Exercises for the Shoulders and Upper Body

The shoulder joint is a ball and socket arrangement in which the humerus of the upper arm fits into the glenoid cavity of the scapula or shoulder blade. The joint does not allow universal movement since it is restricted by supporting structures such as the coracoacromial ligaments. Even without these ligaments, the structure of the shoulder joint allows movement only in a lateral direction up to 90 degrees. For the arm to be raised above the head, joints in the upper limb girdle (the acromioclavicular and sternoclavicular joints) work together with the superior joint of the forearm. Thus, for some movements of the arm, the shoulder joint and arm joint must work together with the upper limb girdle.

A major muscle in the upper arm/shoulder is the deltoid muscle which surrounds the lateral, anterior and posterior sides of the shoulder joint. It works mainly during outward lifting and rotational movements of the arm towards the front or rear. Other muscles involved in moving the arm and upper limb girdle include the teres major and teres minor, as well as the infraspinous and supraspinous. Two other powerful muscles involved in shoulder and arm movement connect the midline of the body (spine

The weight machine being used here builds up the entire pectoral area. The dumb-bell flye is an alternative and perhaps more beneficial exercise using free weights.

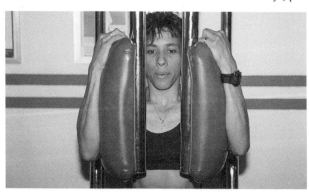

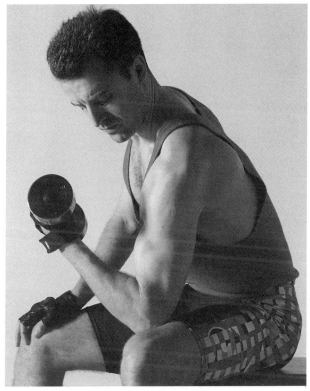

This is a good exercise for the biceps. Grasp the dumb-bell tightly in the left hand, then fully extend the forearm towards the floor. Bring back to the starting position and repeat.

or breast bone) with the upper limb girdle or arm. The pectoral muscle covers the chest, while the trapezius covers the upper back, sweeping up to connect the shoulders and back of the neck with the upper limb girdle. Underneath and just below the trapezius is the latissimus dorsi connecting the upper limb girdle with the lower spine. Two other muscles involved in both neck and shoulder movement are the sternocleidomastoid muscle and the minor pectoral muscle.

Dumb-bell Laterals

+ Stand upright, feet slightly apart, with a dumb-bell in each hand.
+ Hold the arms out from the sides of body, palms of the hands turned in towards the body. Keeping your arms straight, alternately raise your arms, until the weights are level with your ears.
+ Hold briefly before lowering.
+ Do 10 repetitions with weights of 5-7 kg (10-15 lb).

Bent-Over Lateral Raise

+ Sit at one end of a bench with a dumb-bell in each hand.
+ Bend at the waist, lowering the dumb-bells to the ankles. Keeping the arms straight, lift the weights out and up to each side in as wide an arc as possible.
+ Throughout the exercise remain bending.
+ Do 10 repetitions with weights of 5-7 kg (10-15 lb).

This exercise works the deltoids which enclose the shoulder joints.

Dumb-bell Press

+ Standing with a dumb-bell in each hand, hold one in front of the body and the other at your side.
+ Push the one at your side over the head and towards the opposite shoulder.
+ Hold briefly before returning to the starting position. Work this arm 10 times before changing to the other arm.
+ Do 10 repetitions with each arm using 5-7 kg (15-20 lb) weights.

Shoulder Shrug

This movement specifically exercises the trapezius muscle, which covers the upper back and reaches up to connect the shoulders and the back of the neck with the upper limb girdle.

+ Stand upright with your arms straight and hands one shoulder width apart, holding a barbell with an overhand grip.
+ Raise your shoulders as high as possible. Make sure that you keep your arms straight and remain upright throughout the movement.
+ Lower your shoulders to the start position to complete one repetition.
+ Do 10 repetitions with weights of 7-9 kg (15-20 lb).

Seated Dumb-Bell Presses

- Sit at one end of a bench with a dumb-bell in each hand.
- Hold the dumb-bells at shoulder height with palms facing forward.
- Pushing elbows out at the sides, extend both arms upward until at full stretch.

Hold briefly before lowering to the start position. Do 10 repetitions with weights of 5–7 kg (10–15 lb).

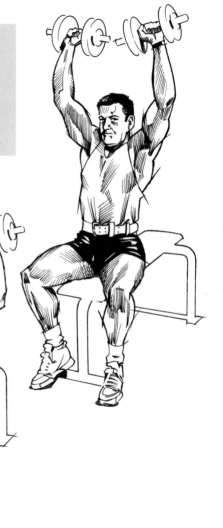

Upright Rows

- Stand with feet one shoulder width apart, holding the barbell at arm's length down in front of the body.
- Keeping the bar as close to the body as possible, lift it smoothly upwards to just below the chin with the elbows out to the sides.
- Do 10 repetitions with weights of 7–9 kg (15–20 lb).

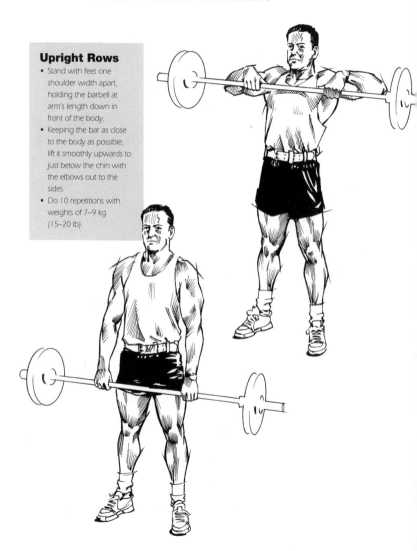

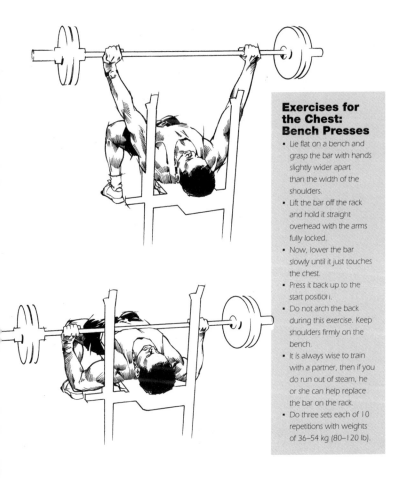

Exercises for the Chest: Bench Presses

- Lie flat on a bench and grasp the bar with hands slightly wider apart than the width of the shoulders.
- Lift the bar off the rack and hold it straight overhead with the arms fully locked.
- Now, lower the bar slowly until it just touches the chest.
- Press it back up to the start position.
- Do not arch the back during this exercise. Keep shoulders firmly on the bench.
- It is always wise to train with a partner, then if you do run out of steam, he or she can help replace the bar on the rack.
- Do three sets each of 10 repetitions with weights of 36–54 kg (80–120 lb).

Dumb-Bell Flyes

- Lie back on the bench with a dumb-bell in each hand.
- Hold them straight overhead with the elbows locked.
- Now, turn the palms inward, bringing the weights together and lower to each side until they are level with the bench.
- Hold for a few moments and then return to the start position.
- Try to keep the weights moving in the same arc and prevent them from drifting in towards the waist.
- Do three sets each of 10 repetitions with 7–9 kg (15–20 lb) weights.

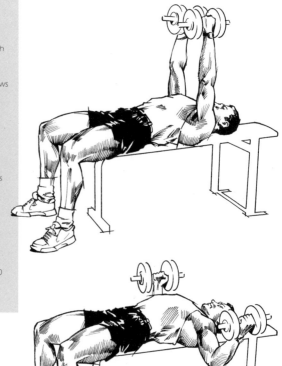

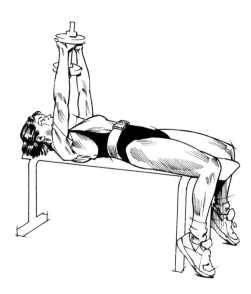

Pullovers

- Lie on the bench and grasp a dumb-bell with both hands.
- Raise it above the chest, then take it over the head and lower it on to the floor behind you. Move the arms in a wide smooth arc, remembering to keep them straight.
- Return to the start position with the dumb-bell over the chest.
- Do 3 sets each of 10 repetitions with 9–14 kg (20–30 lb) weights.

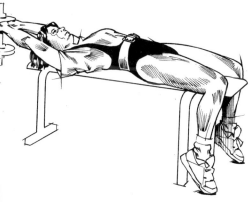

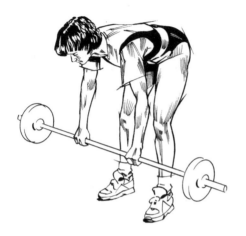

Exercises for the Back: Bent-Over Rows

- Stand in front of the weights, legs one shoulder width apart, and grasp the bar with an overhand grip.
- Rise until the upper body is parallel to the floor. Let the weight hang, keeping the knees slightly bent.
- Now, lift the weight upwards until it just touches the stomach, then lower it slowly. Remain leaning over throughout the exercise and do not rest the weight on the floor between repetitions.
- Do three sets each of 10 repetitions with 11–27 kg (25–60 lb) weights.

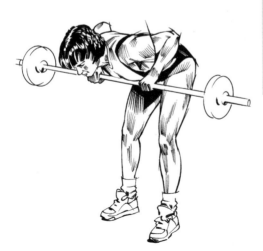

One-Arm Rows

- Pick up a dumb-bell in the left hand and adopt a stance with the left foot forward and the right knee to the rear.
- Bend both knees and lean down until the upper body is parallel with the floor. Let the weight hang free at arm's length. Use the other hand to grasp the edge of the bench for support.
- Now, lift the weight to the side of the chest and lower back again under control.
- Exercise each arm for a full set of 10 repetitions before changing arms.
- Do three sets of 10 repetitions on each arm with 9–14 kg (20–30 lb) weights.

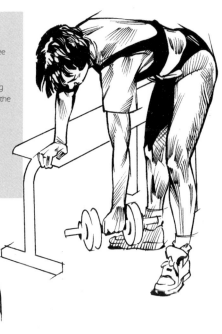

Deadlift

- Stand with your feet one shoulder width apart, then squat down to grasp the bar in front of you. Hold the bar in an overhand grip with one hand and an underhand grip with the other. These two grips will help to maintain balance.
- Keeping your back straight, lift the weight by straightening the legs.
- Shrug your shoulders back, keep your chin up and back arched.
- When lowering, use the legs as much as possible to control the weight.
- Do three sets each of 10 repetitions with 36–45 kg (80–100 lb) weights.

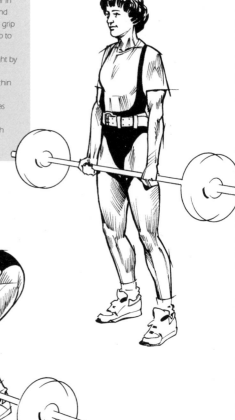

Arm Exercises

The three triceps muscles are located on the back of the upper arm when viewed with the arm held palm uppermost. The large, very obvious muscles at the front of the upper arm, which bulge when the elbow is bent, are the two biceps muscles. These two groups of muscles work antagonistically to flex and straighten the elbow joint.

Below the elbow, the pronator teres muscles and pronator quadratus contract when a person standing with his or her arms at his or her sides rotates the palms towards the rear. Rotation of the palms to the front is controlled by the supinator muscle and the biceps.

This professional weight-lifter reveals the full extent of his biceps muscles in the fully-flexed elbow position. It takes great dedication to build muscle of this stature.

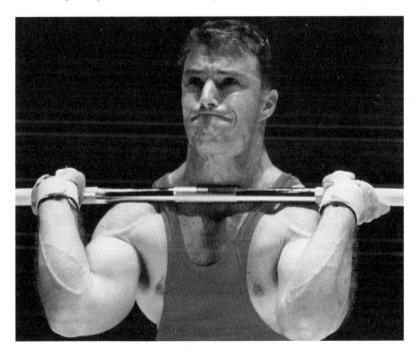

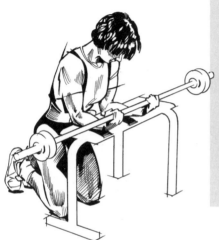

Wrist Curls

- Sit comfortably and grip the bar with palms upward. Bend forward, resting the forearms on the bench with wrists and hands hanging over the edge.
- Bend your wrists, lowering the bar as far as possible towards the ground. When your wrists are bent as far back as they can comfortably go, open your fingers and allow the bar to roll out of your palms.
- Curl the weight back into the palms and flex your hands as high as possible without moving your forearms from the bench.
- Lower the bar again. This completes one repetition. Do three sets each of 10 repetitions with 18–27 kg (40–50 lb) weights.

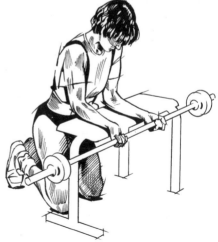

Barbell Curls

- Grasp the barbell with an upward palm grip, hands placed one shoulder width apart.
- Standing comfortably with legs apart, raise the bar and let it hang at arm's length.
- Keeping the elbows fixed, use the lower arms to raise the bar until it just brushes the chin. Hold briefly before lowering again.
- Do three sets of 10 repetitions with 14–20 kg (30–45 lb) weights.

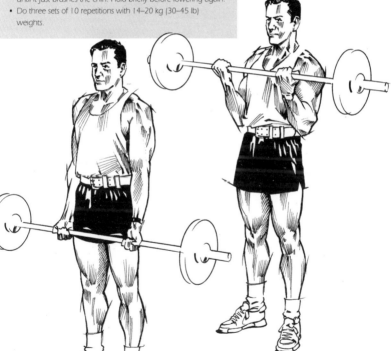

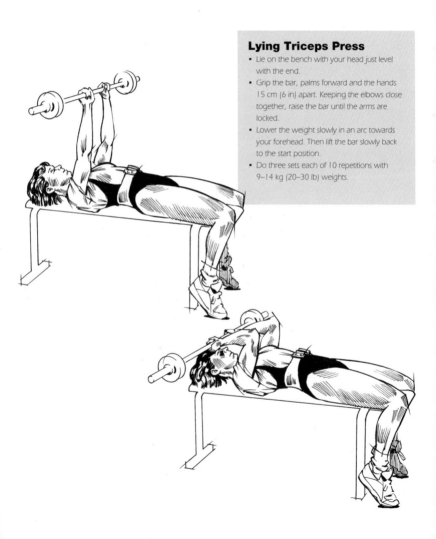

Lying Triceps Press

- Lie on the bench with your head just level with the end.
- Grip the bar, palms forward and the hands 15 cm (6 in) apart. Keeping the elbows close together, raise the bar until the arms are locked.
- Lower the weight slowly in an arc towards your forehead. Then lift the bar slowly back to the start position.
- Do three sets each of 10 repetitions with 9–14 kg (20–30 lb) weights.

Exercising the Buttocks and Lower Legs

Three gluteal muscles stretch from the back of the pelvic girdle to the femur (long bone of the thigh). The largest of these is the gluteus maximus, a strong, thick muscle which forms the majority of the buttocks and works to retract the thigh back in line with the trunk (important when, for example, kicking a ball). This muscle plays an essential role in enabling humans to walk upright. The other two gluteal muscles are used by the body to help support the trunk when standing on one leg.

The action of the gluteus maximus is opposed by the iliopsoas muscles, which flex the hip joint to draw the femur towards the front of the body. Once again, these are antagonistic groups of muscles. The iliopsoas group includes the iliacus muscle which connects the top of the femur to the upper pelvis, and the psoas muscle which runs from the femur to the lumbar spine. These muscles are exercised most effectively by sit-ups.

Other muscles run from the pelvis to attach at varying distances along the femur and the top of the tibia. The job of these long, powerful muscles, such as the sartorius, long abductor muscle and gracilis muscle, is to pull the leg back towards the body but, because of the way they are attached, they also rotate the hip and in some instances the knee. The sartorius, for example, allows us to sit cross-legged.

The group of muscles known as the quadriceps are located at the front of the thigh. They work antagonistically with the biceps at the rear of the thigh. The biceps group, also known as the hamstring, consists of the semimembranosus muscle, semitendinosus muscle and biceps femoris. Together, these two groups of muscles contract to flex the knee joint. When the quadriceps muscles are contracted the leg is extended and when the biceps are contracted the knee is bent.

The gastrocnemius and soleus muscles are found at the back of the calf, the soleus lying somewhat deeper than the larger gastrocnemius. These muscles form a group known as the triceps muscles of the calf. As these muscles run towards the ankle, they form the longest tendon in the body: the Achilles tendon. Their function is to move the ankle joint. These calf muscles are partly opposed by gravity and partly by a series of flexor muscles in the upper part of the foot. Another important muscle involved in lower leg movement is the anterior tibial muscle. This lies just above the tibia bone, which connects the knee to the upper foot.

Squats

- Stand with feet slightly further apart than one shoulder width.
- Grip the bar and balance it across the shoulders, keeping your head and back as straight as possible.
- Now bend your knees and lower your body until your thighs are parallel with the floor. Keep your back straight and eyes fixed on some distant point.
- It is best if you start this exercise with the weights resting on a rack. Have a companion or instructor at hand to help you in case of difficulty.
- Do three sets each of 10 repetitions with 36–45 kg (80–100 lb) weights.

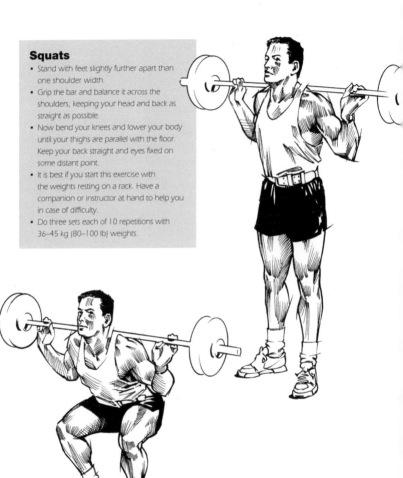

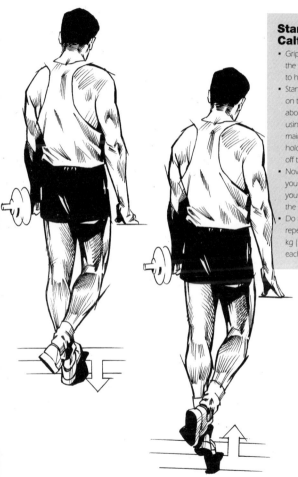

Standing Calf Raises

- Grip the dumb-bell with the left hand and allow it to hang by your side.
- Stand with your right foot on the edge of a platform about 10 cm (4 in) high, using your free hand to maintain balance and holding your right leg just off the ground.
- Now, raise yourself on your toes and then lower your heel until it touches the ground.
- Do three sets each of 20 repetitions with 23–36 kg (50–80 lb) weights for each leg.

Leg Extensions

For this exercise you will need a bench
  equipped with a leg extension machine.

- Sit comfortably on the bench with your feet
  under the padded bar.
- Grip the sides of the bench firmly and
  straighten your legs slowly until they are
  locked.
- Lower slowly back to the starting position.
- Do three sets of 10 repetitions with
  36–45 kg (80–100 lb) weights.

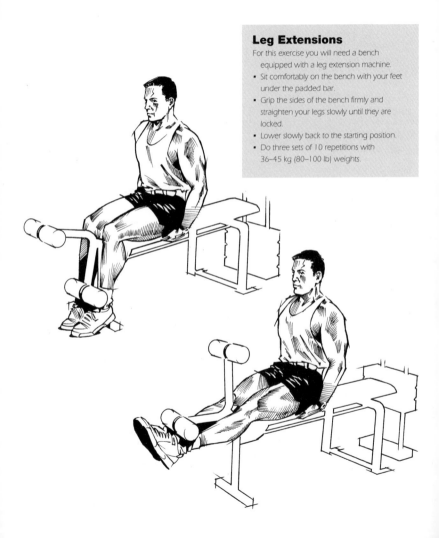

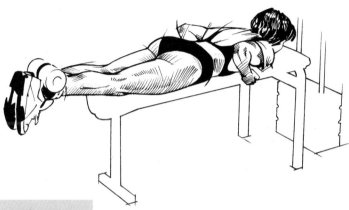

Leg Curls

- Using the same bench, lie face down with ankles hooked under the upper padded bar.
- Holding the bench firmly, curl your legs around the bar until your feet touch your buttocks.
- Do three sets of 10 repetitions with 18–23 kg (40–50 lb) weights.

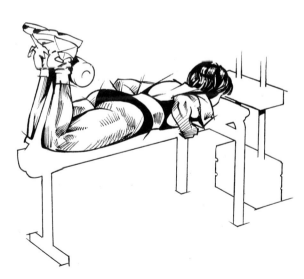

Weight Training Programmes

Initially, we are going to use some of these exercises to work all the muscle groups in turn. As we progress through the programme, we will incorporate the remainder of the exercises into our work-outs and then, finally, we start to use heavier weights. Always keep safety in mind and start with whatever weight feels comfortable.

Novice

WARM-UP	6 MINUTES	
STRETCHING	2 MINUTES	

EXERCISE	REPETITIONS	SETS
DUMB-BELL LATERALS	10	3
FLYES	10	3
BENT-OVER ROWS	10	3
ST. CALF RAISES	10	3
BARBELL CURLS	10	3
SQUATS	5	3
WARM-DOWN		

Once you have mastered this routine, try adding extra weight on the second and third sets. Persevere with the exercises which work the shoulders, chest, back, arms and legs. Because the legs have large, powerful muscles, we exercise them twice. Take a three-minute break between repetitions and a five-minute break between sets.

Intermediate

WARM-UP	**6 MINUTES**
STRETCHING	**2 MINUTES**

EXERCISE	REPETITIONS	SETS
DUMB-BELL LATERALS	10	3
FLYES	10	3
BENT-OVER ROWS	10	3
ST. CALF RAISES	10	3
BARBELL CURLS	10	3
SQUATS	10	3
UPRIGHT ROWS	5	3
BENCH PRESSES	5	3
ONE ARM ROWS	5	3
ST. CALF RAISES	5	3
LYING TRICEPS PRESSES	5	3
SQUATS	5	3
WARM-DOWN		

You must feel comfortable with this training regime before you decide to progress to the advanced programme. By now, you will have a good idea what weight you can manage in each of the exercises. Start the first set of exercises with slightly less weight than the maximum weight you can comfortably manage. On the second set, increase to your maximum comfortable weight and on the last set, try to exceed this weight and do as many repetitions as possible.

Advanced

WARM-UP	6 MINUTES
STRETCHING	2 MINUTES

EXERCISE	REPETITIONS	SETS
DUMB-BELL LATERALS	10	3
UPRIGHT ROWS	10	3
BENT-OVER LATERALS	10	3
DUMB-BELL PRESSES	10	3
BENCH PRESSES	10	3
FLYES	10	3
PULLOVERS	10	3
SQUATS	10	3
ST. CALF RAISES	10	3
LEG EXTENSIONS	10	3
LEG CURLS	10	3
BARBELL CURLS	10	3
LYING TRICEPS PRESSES	10	3
WRIST CURLS	10	3
BENT-OVER ROWS	10	3
ONE ARM ROWS	10	3
DEADLIFTS	10	3
SQUATS	10	3
ST. CALF RAISES	10	3
LEG EXTENSIONS	10	3
LEG CURLS	10	3
WARM-DOWN		

This routine will make you stronger. In order to use this strength to its full advantage, you must incorporate weight training into your long-term training programme, together with circuits, assault courses and running.

Weight Machines

You will find weight machines in most gymnasiums and health centres. These provide us with a useful work-out which can be built in to our overall programme. Although free weights are the better tools in weight training, machines can duplicate many of the pushing/pulling actions. One great advantage of machines is that you can do a number of exercises by just moving a pulley. The resistance – and thus the weight – can be altered by simply moving a pin. Machines do not require you constantly to maintain control or the point of balance that is necessary when working with barbells. Consequently, machines are very safe, allowing an individual the freedom to work on his or her own.

Machines have a different feel to that of free weights and they can give a false impression of what you are achieving, although they are very good for recovery exercises. Other good exercises for machines include seated pull- downs, which work the upper arms, neck and shoulders, and pull-ups, which exercise specific muscles in the arms and shoulders.

Pull-Ups

♦ Stand with legs slightly apart, gripping the bar at waist level.
♦ Raise the bar to the chin with upper arms parallel to the floor.

Standing Pull-Downs

♦ Stand erect with both hands holding the bar.
♦ Pull down to the waist and hold briefly before allowing the bar to rise under control.
♦ Do three sets each of 10 repetitions.

Machines are ideal for these exercises and the only ones that I would recommend. Do three sets each of 10 repetitions. All the other exercises described earlier in this chapter are more effective using free weights.

SAS Weight Training Programme

You should do the advanced programme on alternate days, say Monday, Wednesday and Friday.

Monday: Do the first set of exercises with weights that are comfortable for you. For the next set, add 2–4 kg (5–10 lb). On the last set of exercises, go back to the comfortable weight but add two repetitions to each of

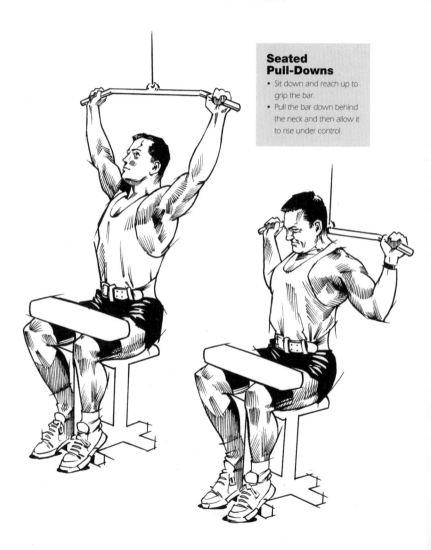

Seated Pull-Downs

- Sit down and reach up to grip the bar.
- Pull the bar down behind the neck and then allow it to rise under control.

the work-outs. Finish the session by burning out the arm muscles, which means doing as many repetitions as possible.

Wednesday: Do Monday's programme in reverse order. Finish by burning out the leg muscles.

Friday: Do the programme with half the weight but do 30 repetitions on the final set of exercises. Next Friday, do 40 repetitions and on the third Friday increase this to 50 repetitions. On the fourth Friday, add 2 kg (5 lb) to all the weights. Now go back to the beginning. Finish each session by burning out the chest muscles with bench presses. You will need a friend to offer encouragement and to recover the weight bar.

Over-Training

Almost any change in personality, habits or mental well-being can indicate over-training. Over-training stresses your body and mind and, perhaps not surprisingly, the signs of over-training are also the symptoms of stress.

1 Loss of appetite
2 Difficulty in getting to sleep or waking unusually early
3 Irritability
4 Difficulty in concentrating
5 Tiredness/mild depression
6 Lack of interest in training
7 Small anxieties or life-stresses which are blown up out of proportion
8 An unusual frequency of minor illnesses such as colds and skin infections

The relationship between mental well-being and performance is so important for professional athletes that sports psychologists use a series of tests to identify and deal with problems. These include the Profile of Mood States (POMS), Sports Competition Anxiety Test (SCAT) and Sport Emotional Reaction Profile (SERP). Do not underestimate the importance of keeping mentally and physically fit or the dangers of over-training. Over-training is more than counter-productive; it can cast a pall over your life. Set reasonable targets and complete the exercises in a time-frame which is realistic for you. Rome was not built in a day and your body will not become stronger overnight. Be patient with your training programme and try not to expect too much too soon. Do not demoralise yourself by continually weighing yourself or getting out the tape measure. You, your training companion and other friends doing the programme will advance at different rates. When your progress seems slow, it is always tempting to over-train by increasing the weight or the number of repetitions. Stick to your own personal programme; it is the only way to make real progress.

Do not be fooled by advertisements in newspapers and magazines offering courses that 'build muscles in weeks'. These are just clever marketing ploys which prey on people's ignorance and fantasies. There are no short cuts. It is hard work, requiring regular training sessions with a range of exercises and lots of self-motivation! At the same time, your fitness programme will help you avoid the other great pitfall of regular training which is obsession. There is always the danger of fitness training taking over your life to the point where all your spare time is spent in the gym. This is not a good thing. You should always work to maintain a balance in your life. How else will you be able to use your new-found strength, stamina and confidence to tackle new challenges?

Fitness can be addictive. Endorphins and other biochemicals are released into the blood during hard, intensive exercise, dampening down pain and producing a 'high'. It is great to get this buzz but it is not worth sacrificing your social life, close friends and family. Exercise and fitness cannot be allowed to take over your life; you have to remain in control.

Equally, pain from torn muscles and other minor injuries should never be ignored. The only way to allow an injury to heal is either to cut down your exercise drastically or stop for a while and seek professional advice.

If your training programme leaves you feeling tired, weak or depressed, it is time either for a change of pace, a different exercise regime or, perhaps, a complete rest. Put quite simply, you have been over-training and this is the body's way of protesting. This is also true of those times when you are no longer enjoying the training or when you are left with the feeling that you are simply not progressing. This is not something which develops in a couple of days; it has probably been building up for months. We cannot allow our bodies and minds to become stale. That is why on the severe SAS programme we build in a break on the sixth training week. This provides a welcome rest and serves to sharpen our appetite to resume training with a vengeance.

Of course, you will experience peaks and troughs in your training routine; this is only natural. Some days you will feel as though you could keep training forever but on other days it will be an effort just to put the weights on the bar. When you start getting more 'bad' days than 'good' ones, ask yourself if you are over-training. If the answer is yes, then get out of the gym and go and read a book or lie in the sun. Playing with your children, kicking a ball around or weeding the garden are also forms of exercise but it is the type of exercise that rejuvenates. Psychiatrists call it 'masterful inactivity'. Very soon you will be able to return to the gym fully revitalised. However, if, as soon as you walk in the gym door, your enthusiasm starts to wane again, maybe it is time to change training facilities. Perhaps the other clients are getting on your nerves or there is insufficient support from the staff or the apparatus is old and is out of order more times than it is in use. Try working out amongst different faces; new people will freshen your mind.

You will soon become aware of the changes in your physical and mental abilities. You will become aware of your body's potential. You will also learn about your body's limitations and be able to tailor these to your personal fitness programme. The right combination of exercises and regular work-outs will enable you to develop a natural instinct for what is right for you as an individual.

Having said so much about over-training, perhaps I ought to say a little about how you should be able to feel and behave when training is going well and you are riding the crest of the wave of achievement and self-fulfilment.

1   You should be able to concentrate totally throughout an entire training session.
2   You should be able to put more effort and intensity into the exercises as you progress through the programme.
3   Your confidence should allow you to perform up to expectation.
4   You should be able to identify and work on weaknesses and plan further training schedules.
5   Small life-stresses and anxieties should not affect your training.
6   A 'bad' training session should not destroy your confidence.
7   You should know how to train to regain lost confidence.
8   You should maintain the willpower to excel and improve.

Isometrics

Another method of strength training is through the use of isometric exercises. This involves pushing and pulling against objects that cannot move, such that the muscles are made to work with the minimum of contraction. The main disadvantage is that strength gains tend to be limited to the limb position and angle used in training. In isometric regimes, strength gains are seen after five to six weeks when 10 repetitions (each lasting at least six seconds) of the exercise are repeated three times per week.

Focusing the Mind

It is important to be able to focus the mind, enabling you to concentrate on the matter in hand. Equally, it is important to clear your mind of the many distractions of everyday living so that you can focus your entire concentration on the training ahead. The following exercise is designed to do just that and should be used just prior to your warm-up. Stand erect but relaxed with feet one shoulder width apart. Mentally picture your body and start to relax.

Beginning at your head, imagine that you are forcing all the tension down your body to 'escape' through your shoe-laces. Close your eyes and deal with the tension in your forehead and sides of the face. You should feel your head getting lighter. In your mind's eye, suck the tension inwards and channel it downwards. Relax the neck and let the shoulders slump. Next, relax your arms. They should start to become heavier as the muscles no longer fight against gravity. Breathe easily, slackening the chest, back, stomach and buttocks. Imagine that you are breathing from the very core of your body.

Relax the knees and imagine that they are oak trees with roots spreading down into the soil. Clear your mind of worries and start to think positively as to what you are about to achieve. Take your time. You should now be relaxed. It does not matter if you sway a little; even oak trees do that!

Weight Training Routines

To be frank, you really need the services of a well-equipped gym for weight training. Working out at home with limited equipment, and without a companion or instructor to offer encouragement, is obviously less than ideal. In a gym, you will meet other experienced athletes who can offer encouragement and show you what you can achieve with time and training. Strike up a friendship with a more experienced person using the gym. It is good to train with someone stronger, faster and fitter than yourself. It is the same with any sport. By playing with a superior opponent who is more intense, driving you forward and always offering you encouragement, your game is much more likely to improve. Later, when you are more experienced, the opportunity will undoubtedly present itself for you to offer the same support to another novice. As the well-known maxim reminds us: what comes around, goes around.

Heavy Training Routines

Try this routine to increase strength and build muscle. It consists of five sets of exercises. The work-out begins with a high number of repetitions which decrease with each set of exercises, but to compensate we increase the weight each time.

Set No 1 - 15 repetitions with 36 kg (80 lb)
Set No 2 - 10 repetitions with 41 kg (90 lb)
Set No 3 - 8 repetitions with 45 kg (100 lb)
Set No 4 - 6 repetitions with 50 kg (110 lb)
Set No 5 - 4 repetitions with 54 kg (120 lb)

These are only suggested weights in order to demonstrate the general idea. Choose your own weights and, if you become exhausted before the last set, modify the programme by decreasing the number of repetitions in each set. Try to finish with the highest weight that you can safely manage. You will need to do at least three to five complete sets if you are to see any benefit. Remember to rest between each set in order to give your muscles time to recover. This routine will build muscle but it will be at the expense of speed.

High Intensity Training

This type of routine offers only the minimum rest time between each set of exercises. It is excellent for developing speed and endurance. The idea is that you try to work as hard as you can for as long as you are able. We call this 'rapid heart exertion'. This is the very essence of fitness training, doing as much as possible in a given time. To use an analogy, it is the difference between running and jogging. When jogging, you may cover 4 km (2½ miles) in, say, 50 minutes. Your stride is short and leg-lift is minimal, and the heart and lungs are not unduly exerted. In contrast, during a 50-minute run you cover twice that distance, and heart and lungs will have to work much harder. The same principle is used in high-intensity weight training. Use moderately heavy weights and go through the work-out as fast as possible. The danger here is taking short cuts. You need to stay focused, doing the full range of movements and controlling the weights at all times.

Low Repetition Training

Low repetition training is ideal for the older person who is seeking greater mobility. By doing a few repetitions with light to average weights, he or she can go through the full range of movements that they would normally find hard to achieve. Weights are an excellent exercise for this purpose, and after a low repetition session a feeling of elation is experienced.

Free Weights v Machines

Most gyms have both machines and free weights, and these can be combined in your work-out programme. Free weights are, of course, more tricky to use since they must be controlled at all times. Machine weights are only lifted and controlled in the vertical plane; the weight cannot get out of control and the worst that can happen is that it will fall with an almighty crash. As I have mentioned previously, machines do have one serious disadvantage in that they can give a false impression of power. The power needed to raise a 45 kg (100 lb) weight on a machine may, in real terms, only be equal to that required to raise a 36 kg (80 lb) free weight.

That said, it is useful to mix the two in your work-out. In particular, cycling, skiing and rowing machines are a good way of warming up and warming down. Treadmills, which can be set at various speeds, can also be integrated into your programme. Treadmills are particularly good for warming down. Over a six-minute period, you can gradually reduce the speed until your heart beat and respiration return to normal. One disadvantage is that the treadmill is always in demand in a gym and the staff and other clients will take a dim view of the matter if you hog it to run a marathon!

Weight and Machine Routine

W = weights **M** = mach ne

CYCLE	6 MINUTES	

	EXERCISE	REPETITIONS	SETS
M	FLYES	10	3
M	CALF RAISES	10	3
M	PULL-DOWNS	10	3
W	LEG CURLS	10	3
W	UPRIGHT ROWS	10	3
W	LATERAL RAISES	10	3
M	TRICEPS PUSH-DOWNS	10	3
W	BENCH PRESSES	10	3
M	LEG EXTENSIONS	10	3
W	ARM EXTENSIONS	10	3
M	LEG CURLS	10	3
W	PULLOVERS	10	3

TREADMILL	6 MINUTES	

The leg extension and leg curl machines mentioned earlier provide excellent remedial exercise to help you overcome certain types of injuries and are often recommended by physiotherapists.

Machines also offer the novice a very easy way into weight training and an easy progression to free weights. Of course, much more care is required with barbells and dumb-bells. I have seen weights that have not been secured correctly fall off, causing injury. There was also the occasion when a sudden shifting of the point of balance detached a weight from a barbell, resulting in quite a severe injury.

Let us now have a look at a simple programme which offers a combination of machine and free-weight exercises. This routine exercises all the important muscle groups and should take you around 45 minutes to complete. I use this work-out frequently, sometimes adding repetitions to burn out the arm or leg muscles in the last set.

CHAPTER FOUR

Running

Running is the basis of all fitness. It is a vital part of many sports and games and, as part of a fitness programme, has no equal.

Let us set the record straight. There is a big difference between running and jogging. You could jog until your legs ached and your feet blistered and still not gain any real long-term benefit.

In contrast, running conditions the heart and lungs for speed and endurance. It requires no special equipment, it can be done at any time of the day and it is absolutely free.

Choose a route that is quiet and avoids major roads. In particular, avoid heavy traffic since the danger from pollution outweighs the benefits gained from the exercise. Running can be boring, so a scenic route is best; looking at stimulating countryside helps pass the time. When the route starts to resemble an old television film, run in the reverse direction or choose a number of different routes. Try to include some hills in the run, since these will enable you to develop strength and stamina more rapidly.

Some Problems

By following a few simple rules, the disadvantages of running can be minimised. Blisters are easily avoidable as long as we take care of our feet

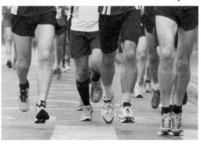

and select the right socks and running shoes (or boots!). You do not need fancy, expensive trainers. In the SAS, we ran and trained in boots. There were no 'go faster' shoes available for the deserts and jungles in which we operated. Heavy footwear gives a harder work-out and also protects feet from heavy pounding on hard surfaces. Damage to muscles and tendons, and the more serious stress

Make sure you wear well-fitting and sturdy running shoes for running to avoid undue discomfort to your feet. Blisters are painful and take quite a while to heal.

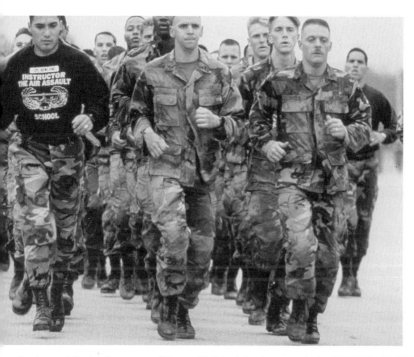

fractures of the leg bones, can all be avoided by following a gradual programme. Such damage is usually due to over-training – doing too much too soon.

Action

Running is a natural activity which everyone can enjoy. It is an excellent way of clearing the mind of all your daily woes and should be regarded as a treat rather than a chore. The secret is to relax. Avoid tension in your arms and shoulders, lean forward slightly and choose a long, comfortable stride. Keep your arms relaxed with hands slightly clenched, thumbs

Follow the experts' example and get into a relaxed, comfortable stride when running. Do not tense your arms or flex the knees but aim for a long and low leg movement.

uppermost. An easy rhythmic arm motion helps to maintain momentum and balance. Do not flex the knee more than is necessary. Sprinters need to raise their knees to gain speed but a low, wide stride is more useful for covering long distances.

Distance

We are going to introduce different running programmes for specific training requirements. The intensity of the run is more important than the distance. Generally, speed is built up by short, fast runs, while long-distance runs develop endurance.

First Steps

Find a time of day when you have a spare 30 minutes. Evenings and

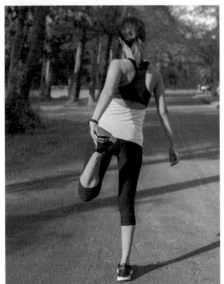

early mornings may offer the best window in a busy schedule. Select a 5-km (3-mile) circuit and jog for as long as possible. When you can jog no longer, cover the ground with a fast walk. Use the walking phases to allow your body to recover and then move back into a jogging pace.

Run on alternate days and soon the 5-km (3-mile) circuit will offer no more challenges. Once you find this happening, try to run the circuit in a faster time. A cheap stop-watch will help you keep track of your personal times. Break the run with short, fast sprints, followed by an easy jog to recover. Practice exaggerating your stride and knee-lift; you are looking for an even pace of about 10 km/h (6 miles per hour). This easy pace will enable you to cover quite long distances quickly. Heavily laden soldiers in some regiments use this technique to cover ground. In the Second World War, it was known as the 'Commando Trot'.

Short Run
The next step is to cover a fairly flat, 5-km (3-mile) circuit in 30 minutes. Sprint the last 100 m (100 yds).

Fun Run
This should last for an hour and cover about 8.5 km (5 miles). Include a few hills as a hedge against boredom. Again, sprint the last 100 m (100 yds).

Fast Run
Run the 5-km (3-mile) circuit as fast as you can manage. Set yourself the task of beating your best personal time.

Long Run
Now you are ready for the long run: a 16-km (10-mile) route in 90 minutes. Choose a scenic route with plenty of gradients. Start slowly and finish strongly. Sprint the last 100 m (100 yds).

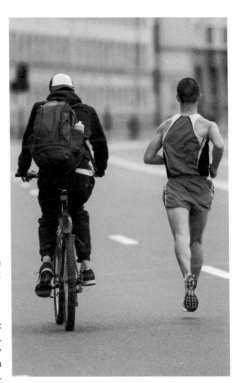

Try a long-distance run in conjunction with a training partner on a cycling session. He or she can carry supplies of food and drink, and you can spur each other on.

Some Useful Advice
Some dogs like chasing runners. They are just playing, but they can be a nuisance. If the runner becomes aggressive or obviously shows fear, the encounter can turn nasty. Stand still, protect the area of your groin, avoid eye contact with the animal and, speaking gently but firmly, command him to 'sit' or 'stay'. Finally, walk away calmly. Ensure that you are some distance away from the animal before continuing your run.

CHAPTER FIVE

Endurance Marches

The hallmark of the Special Forces is the ability, if necessary, to move long distances every day for the duration of their mission. Frequently, they will be carrying the entire equipment for their mission – often as much as 68 kg (150 lb) of gear. It is not unusual for an SAS exercise to begin with a 65-km (40-mile) infiltration, which will be completed in as little as nine hours. To select the men with the right calibre, a selection course was devised which took the candidates to the limits of their endurance. Under great physical and mental hardship, it was reasoned, the men's true nature would be revealed. Those with the 'right stuff' kept themselves going, while accurately navigating from rendezvous to rendezvous (RV). But there was more. Throughout this ordeal, they had to keep functioning as prospective SAS soldiers, remembering their RV drills and watching and memorising the changing landscape. Many people have asked me the secret of passing SAS selection. There is no secret and there are no short-cuts. It is hard work and you simply have to want it enough. There is only one way to carry a pack long distances and that is to simply get up and do it.

Rucksack

Once you have shouldered your pack, it must be forgotten. However, you can only do this if the pack is comfortable.

Select a pack that suits you. There is an excellent range of good military and mountaineering/hill-walking packs available from shops specialising in outdoor activity equipment. Yes, of course, some of them will be very expensive but the time and effort spent producing the top commercial packs more than justifies the price tag. A good rucksack should last a lifetime.

When choosing a pack, look carefully at its suspension system. Ensure that the pack has well-padded straps that are fully adjustable. A padded hip belt takes a lot of the strain off the shoulders. Heavy packs can cause

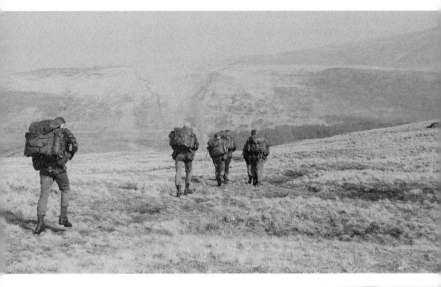

bruising and chafing of the shoulders. The rucksack should have a good frame and ample capacity for your needs. A small day pack will have a capacity of around 20 litres (3 cubic feet), whereas large expedition packs should have a capacity of around 100 litres (42 cu ft). It is better to choose a pack that is too big for your needs than too small. You cannot crush 30 litres (12 cu ft) of kit into a 20-litre (8 cu-ft) pack. On the other hand, if the pack is larger than you need, you do not have to fill it up!

External pockets are very important, since you do not want to be constantly opening the pack and rifling through the contents, particularly when the weather is bad.

The pack should be composed of a strong, long-lasting material such as canvas, and should be supported by a strong frame. This should be recessed or padded so that it does not chafe your back. If you find that areas of the pack are chafing you during walks, these can usually be 'softened' with foam rubber kept in place with electrical tape. Some SAS

SAS soldiers on a long-range endurance march in South Wales. They are well wrapped-up against the elements and carry everything they will need in their bergens.

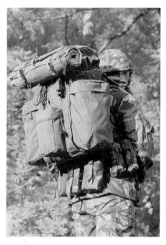

A good rucksack is a vital piece of kit for an endurance march. Choose a modern, high-quality pack that sits high on the shoulders and has external pockets.

men make a rubber pad for their Bergen which is secured over the frame. This can be made from little more than a thin, foam-rubber chair cushion covered in strong polythene.

Check the centre of gravity of your prospective pack. Modern packs have a high centre of gravity, riding high on the shoulders but still contouring the back. The pack should not be too high or it will force you to lean forward and, if caught by the wind, it will transform you into a sailing ship! This becomes extremely important in the mountains, where paths cross steep gradients and winds can reach 97 km/h (60 mph).

Many people buy military-style packs. Certainly, these are often well-designed and have many of the advantages of the more expensive mountaineering packs. However, we should say a few words here on what to avoid. The old 'commando packs', such as the bergen, were originally designed for ski troops and therefore have a low centre of gravity. Most of the weight is carried around the lower back which can lead to spinal problems and terrible 'bergen scars' where the pack has chafed or cut the skin. These packs are now mostly found in army surplus shops – avoid them! Quite apart from the unfortunate design, they tend to have a much smaller capacity than other packs of their size.

The famous SAS bergen is, perhaps, another piece of kit to avoid. Because it serves as a personal parachute container, it comes with a reinforced frame which adds a lot of weight. Unless you are planning to parachute into the gym, it may be better to select a lighter pack! The Cyclops series, used by many Royal Marine Commandos, offers the same advantages but with much lighter frames.

Packing your Rucksack

Do not make the mistake of using sand or bricks to bring your pack up to the required weight. Bricks can damage the pack and sand is a dead weight which will fall to the bottom of the pack, placing undue stress on the spine. Fill your rucksack with useful equipment. You may be grateful to have bad-weather kit or the necessities for making a cup of tea at some point. And if you do sustain an injury out on the hills, you will have all the necessary gear to make yourself comfortable until help arrives. How to pack your Bergen correctly is the first lecture the prospective SAS soldier is given. Weight should be distributed evenly throughout the pack. Start by putting in the kit those items which you will rarely use, or perhaps only once a day, then pack your sleeping bag wrapped in a waterproof bag. A wet sleeping bag is very uncomfortable; it is not efficient at trapping body heat and it can precipitate serious illnesses such as hypothermia.

Next, put in a change of clothing, including boots or trainers. These, too, are wrapped in their own waterproof bag. Remember, packs are water resistant but rarely waterproof! Next comes your tent, a first-aid kit and any other equipment you might need. Try and remember where everything has been placed. You do not really want to keep emptying the pack every time you need a piece of kit.

Under the top flap, carry a set of waterproofs. These should only be worn when resting or doing light work. You can become drenched in sweat very quickly inside waterproofs, and life-threatening hyperthermia is a real possibility if you start to overheat. What is more, the straps of your rucksack will rub the shoulders and the garment will start to leak.

The external pockets are for the equipment that you will use regularly, such as cooking kit, food, water, sweets – in fact everything that you want close to hand.

Clothing

It is important to wear the correct clothing when training. Carrying a pack is hard work so do not over-dress. Wear a cotton T-shirt under a pullover. If the weather is wet or cold, you can wear a windproof smock over the top. The secret to keeping warm is dressing in layers. As the body starts to warm up, peel off the outermost layers and stow them in your pack. Windproof trousers are another good idea, particularly in bad weather. These are worn over your walking trousers or shorts. Finally, you will need well-fitting boots and cotton socks to minimise blisters.

The exertion will make you sweat heavily. Once warm, try not to let your body cool down. Keep your rest-stops to a minimum (five or ten minutes every hour) and put on warm clothing when you stop. Remove the extra layers prior to resuming the march.

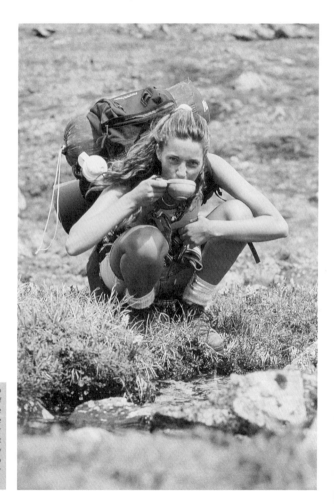

Make sure you keep up your intake of fluids on endurance marches, but take care what you drink. Water from even the clearest mountain stream may be contaminated, so always sterilize water before drinking.

Boots

Choose your boots carefully and be prepared to dip into your pocket. They must be well-fitting and comfortable, waterproof and strong. Look for a boot which gives good ankle support but is not so high as to put strain on the Achilles tendon. Avoid the speed-lacing system since this can snag on undergrowth and cause falls. The laces can also work loose and trip you up.

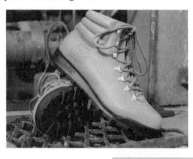

Modern boots break in easily but it still requires some effort on your part. The easiest way to break in boots is to sit in a comfortable chair, with your booted feet in a bowl of water. Leave them immersed for about 30 minutes and then go for a walk. Let them dry naturally. Never place wet boots in front of the fire or a radiator, since this will dry and crack the leather.

Do not skimp on the quality of boots you purchase for endurance marches. These are ideal, being nicely padded and high enough to give support to the ankle.

Hats

Hats are useful for minimising heat loss. As much as 40 per cent of the heat radiating from the human body is lost from the head and neck. If it is hot, you can always take your hat off and slip it in your pocket. In really cold weather, a woollen ski balaclava is a good piece of kit.

Personal Kit

Personal kit should meet your own particular requirements but should usually include a detailed map of the area and a compass, as well as a small survival kit carried in the breast pocket. A survival knife and change for the telephone (or a phone card) are also important.

Belt Kit

Belt kit is useful, particularly if you are injured or if, for some reason, you have to ditch your rucksack. It should consist of a water bottle and at least one pouch containing some snacks. This way, you will be able to eat and drink on the move.

Starting Out

Now that we have our kit and clothing sorted out we can start training.

Adjust the weight of your pack to around 18 kg (40 lb) - it is difficult to get under this weight if you are carrying the right equipment - and use a park or other open space to get used to the feel of it. Do not start on roads, since pounding on a hard surface may cause foot and leg injuries. Staying close to home, walk around for an hour. Check that your rucksack is properly centred and the straps well-adjusted.

Your first real walks should last about four hours, during which you should aim to cover as much ground as possible. Try to stay off the roads as much as possible. Use the map to select a circuit across open country that will finally take you back home or to your car. Hills, mountains or moorland are ideal, but if you do not have easy access to these, check your Ordnance Survey map for footpaths; once outside the city or town, the countryside is criss-crossed with paths.

When climbing hills, take a shorter step and try to keep going until you reach the summit. When you arrive at the top, lengthen your stride and cover the level ground as quickly as possible. When going downhill, get a firm grip of the pack and move into an easy jog. However, the type of ground and the weight of the pack will determine the maximum safe speed when descending.

The SAS man will cover ground at a steady pace of about 6.5 kmph (4 mph) and 9.5-11 kmph (6-7 mph) when under time pressure. Allow yourself five or ten-minute breaks every hour. It is possible to cover up to 20 km (12¹₂ miles) across rough, mountainous country in four hours. Make this your first target, although it may take many navigation walks before you reach this standard! Once you are familiar with the route, the march will become easier and your best personal time will decrease.

More Advanced Walks

Once you have mastered the 20-km (12¹₂-mile) endurance march, start to increase the weight of your pack. Do this in 2 or 2.5-kg (5 or 10-lb) increments but keep within the four hour time limit. When your rucksack has reached 25 kg (55 lb), aim to cover 40 km (25 miles). With practice, you should be able to cover this in six to eight hours.

At around 32 km (20 miles), you may well find that you 'hit the wall'. This is an expression used by marathon and ultra-marathon runners to denote a state where you start to slow down, your concentration begins to lapse (you may think only of food) and you feel awful. The reason is simple:

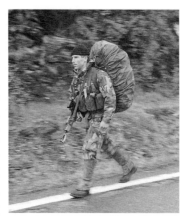

you have run out of fuel. Put quite simply, it takes around 700 g (25 oz) of sugar to cover 40 km (25 miles), and this calculation has been arrived at by studying fuel-efficient, well-conditioned athletic bodies. Even if you have stuffed yourself full of *Mars* bars or potatoes before the walk, 700 g (25 oz) of sugar is much more than all the sugar in the blood and the muscles combined. When your body runs out of sugar, it begins to burn fat; this is burnt much more slowly than sugar and so your performance starts to fall off. Of course, the answer is obvious. Carry some sugar-rich foods, such as *Mars* bars and glucose sweets, and start to consume them steadily once you have passed the half-way point. This will give the sugar time to get into your blood before you start to run out of energy.

An SAS soldier often carries a pack weighing some 68 kg (150 lb). With greater experience, increase the weight you carry while decreasing the distance you cover.

You may find that you also have another problem. As you sweat you will lose salts, resulting in painful muscle cramps. Sweat contains sodium, potassium and chloride ions. These perform much the same function in the body as the electrolytes in a car battery. In days gone by, the British Army issued salt (sodium chloride) tablets to its soldiers, but here is the rub. The normal diet contains more than sufficient sodium unless you are doing an ultra-marathon or the final SAS navigation walks in summer. What is in short supply, and not easily replaced, is potassium. The answer is simple. Carry some juicy, ripe fruit with you. Fruit juice and fruits (particularly bananas) are rich in this mineral.

Once you have completed an eight-hour march with 25 kg (55 lb), you can start to be more ambitious. As with weight training, what we should do now is decrease the distance and increase the weight. An SAS soldier often carries as much as 68 kg (150 lb) on his back.

Try carrying a 36 kg (80 lb) pack for an hour, then with each new session add an hour until you can carry 36 kg (80 lb) for four hours. The pace will be a lot slower but the principle remains the same. Continue with the same hourly rest breaks but try to take them after a particularly demanding section of the route. Increase the weight until you can carry 45 kg (100 lb) for four hours. After carrying a heavy pack, go back to a weight of 25 kg (55 lb) and you will find the difference remarkable. You will feel as though you are flying across the ground.

The SAS Endurance March

On selection for the 22 SAS Regiment, the final navigation march requires you to complete a 60-km (37-mile) route over the Welsh mountains (or similar country), while carrying a 25-kg (55-lb) pack, rifle and belt kit. The time allowed is 20 hours. On this sort of march, you certainly have to pay attention to all the minor details. Good balance is particularly important if you want to conserve your energy. Of course, balance is also essential for safety, particularly on the high mountain paths. The American Indians used to practice walking with their toes pointed slightly inward. If you let the toes point outward, it becomes difficult to walk in a straight line. Equally, try to avoid walking on your heels since this also unbalances the body. It is better to lean forward into your line of march than backwards. A slight roll of the shoulders also helps with momentum. Walk in such a way that your entire foot makes contact with the ground. This way, the body's weight is evenly distributed which is very important when carrying heavy loads. Do not try to walk on your toes since this irritates the Achilles tendon and the connecting calf muscles. When climbing straight up steep slopes, you should use only your toes. An alternative is to climb very steep gradients on a diagonal route or zig-zag up the hill, resting where necessary. Just a brief halt for 30 or 40 seconds is all that is required to let the leg muscles recover. A diagonal climb also allows you to put as much of your foot on the ground as possible. Although it will require more energy to climb the hill this way, the overall effort is less demanding. Watch the ground and avoid treading on rocks or loose scree. On the mountains, which get more rain than the lowlands, the rocks can be slippery or may be easily dislodged. Plan your route up the hillside but be prepared to modify it constantly. In particular, keep clear of thick vegetation, rocky outcrops and scree slopes.

Keep out of rivers and streams; they can be difficult to cross and the water may be very fast and very cold. If faced with crossing a fast stream, move further uphill along its banks until the stream narrows sufficiently to effect a safe crossing.

Watch where you place your feet and make sure that every foot-hold is secure before transferring your weight. This becomes particularly important when climbing steep ground. The knee is a very vulnerable joint and an unexpected slip can twist it, causing extensive damage. Once you have gained the summit of the hill, try to work the adjoining ridges and hills into your route and stay on the high ground for as long as possible.

Before leaving the high ground, make very sure that you know your location and that you have chosen the correct route. On very difficult ground (the mountainous jungles of south-east Asia spring to mind) the only way to travel is to climb spurs, walk along the ridge lines and down another spur that corresponds with your line of march. There are few vantage points and all the terrain looks the same. A simple mistake in leaving the high ground on the wrong spur can be disastrous, costing the patrol many hours, sometimes days, of extra walking.

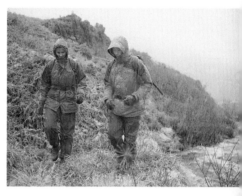

Encourage a friend to accompany you on your marches and take it in turns to lead and set the pace. Plan emergency RVs in case you become separated along the route.

When going downhill, use a short, springy step to control your momentum and jog down the slope. On steep gradients, dig your heels in and use your arms to maintain balance. Never walk with your hands in your pockets. Take care to keep your speed under control. If you find yourself overbalancing or losing control of your speed, lean back and sit down. Back on the flat, use a long, comfortable stride. Try to cover as much ground as possible with each stride. Watch the landscape and note those areas of natural shelter, in case the weather takes a change for the worse. In mountainous terrain, a light, misty rainfall in the valleys can quickly give way to snow on the tops.

Try to take the shortest route possible, although it will sometimes be difficult to march on a straight line and you will have to detour around obstacles. If you go left around one obstacle, go right around the next; with very little effort, this will keep you close to your intended track.

Read the ground and compare the low and high ground to the map contours. When in doubt, use your compass to check the direction of your march. Always trust your compass.

CHAPTER SIX

Swimming

Water is the most powerful element on this planet and must be treated with respect. Every SAS soldier must be confident in the water and the Regiment spends a lot of time ensuring that everyone is up to the required standard. Each squadron has an Amphibious Troop, trained in diving, canoeing and the use of small boats, and troop members must undergo additional training. The annual SAS swimming test is 40 lengths of the baths, wearing trousers and shirt, with a full water bottle attached to a belt. This test must be completed in 50 minutes.

Swimming is also an excellent way of maintaining fitness while recovering from an injury since the water supports the body's weight. Swimming should be included in all fitness schedules as a rest/fun period. Although we can work hard at swimming, it must be enjoyable if it is to break the monotony of a vigorous training programme.

Swimming exercises all of the body with much less exertion on the heart and lungs (swimming is recommended for asthmatics since it is one of the few exercises that does not provoke exercise-induced asthma). So, to get a good work-out from swimming, we need to do some fast laps and relatively long distances.

Starting
If you are a non-swimmer, get down to the baths and take some lessons. There is no quicker way to learn than taking lessons from a qualified instructor. If you intend to spend a lot of time in water, invest in a pair of swimmer's goggles. These will protect your eyes from the chlorine in the water, which can cause quite severe eye irritation. The two basic swimming strokes are breast stroke and front crawl.

Breast Stroke
This is the most economical method of moving through the water. Try to make each stroke as long as possible and glide through each movement.

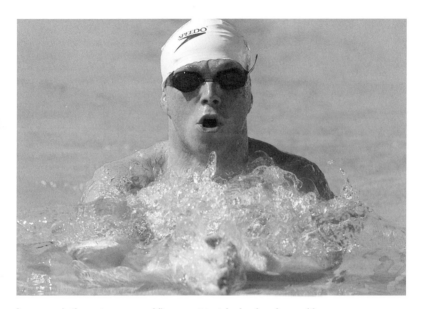

Lay prone in the water, arms and fingers outstretched, palms down with the index fingers touching. The head should be slightly raised with the eyes looking across the surface.

Push off with the legs, keeping their action synchronised. The arms should be about 23 cm (9 in) under the water and held straight. This makes it easier to lift the chest out of the water to breathe. Slide forward and, as your body loses forward momentum, sweep your arms in a wide, powerful arc to regain speed.

As the legs follow through their stroke and relax, inhale, cup the hands and sweep the arms backwards through the water. Ensure that this is a full, powerful stroke that travels all the way back to the thighs. As the arms bend for their recovery stroke, the knees should be bent outwards in readiness for the next kick. Breathe out as the explosive kick straightens the legs and brings them together.

Swimming plays a relatively small but important part in our fitness programme both as an excellent all-round exercise and a respite from more arduous activities.

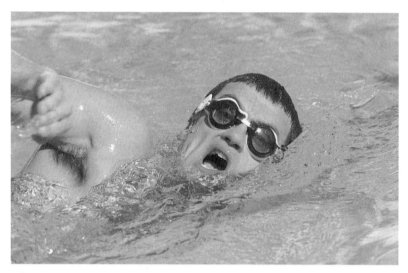

Front crawl is a fast stroke, but the technique takes some time to master. The swimmer should kick the legs six times for every complete cycle of the arms.

The actions on the breast stroke should be graceful and smooth. If it feels jerky, then the motions of the arms and legs are not co-ordinated. The body should continue to glide through the water, in-between the leg and arm actions. As you become more confident, try to breathe only on every second stroke since this is more energy efficient.

Front Crawl

You must decide to which side you prefer to turn your head in order to breathe. Keep your head down and lift your arm clear of the water. Kick using a strong, paddling motion with legs straight. Reach your arm forward then pull it back, holding as much water as possible. Turn your head and take a breath. Lift the other arm clear of the water. As it begins its backward stroke, the first arm is brought forward again. After turning your head to take a breath, you should turn it to the front and exhale under water. Some expert swimmers breathe on every second or third cycle of the arms only. Technique is vital with this stroke if the swimmer is to turn all the available energy into speed. There should be a slight hollow in the back and the forehead should cut through the water, with the eyes just below the surface.

The leg movement is from the hips (not from the knees) in a powerful up and down motion. The legs should be relaxed and slightly bent at the knees. The more flexible and relaxed the movement, the more effective the stroke.

The arms sweep back alternatively, with one pulling as the other recovers. The hand should enter the water on its own side of the centre line approximately between the eye and the shoulder. The arm slightly bent at the elbow presses down on the water and bears downward and backward until the thumb brushes the thigh. This is the signal for the other arm to begin its stroke. The shoulders should remain square during the arm movement.

The most common mistake made with this technique is excessive rolling. This is caused by over-reaching with the arms. This, in turn, is partly due to weak leg actions, such that the arms are trying to work too quickly to propel the body through the water. If the feet come out of the water, the knees are probably bent too much, resulting in shallow leg movements.

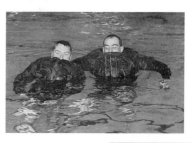

Other Strokes

The back stroke is a useful stroke when tired. If you need a rest, or feel cramp developing, roll on to your back and take a breather. In the military, we spent a lot of time swimming on our backs wearing diver's fins. This is an excellent exercise for the legs. Other strokes, such as the Butterfly and the Dolphin, are very fast, very tiring and require a high standard of training. They cannot be maintained for long periods but are excellent for short, fast bursts of swimming. An ideal way to finish a swim!

Never take water safety lightly. The majority of drownings in fresh water occur within 3 metres (10 ft) of the water's edge and safety. Practice the H.E.L.P. position.

Fun Swim

A 30-minute swim, with alternate lengths doing breast stroke and front crawl, would be a welcome addition to our training programme. Try to do as many lengths in the time as possible.

Breast Stroke

Aim for a good swimming rhythm, correct breathing, relaxation of the legs after the kick-back and good synchronisation between the left and right movements.

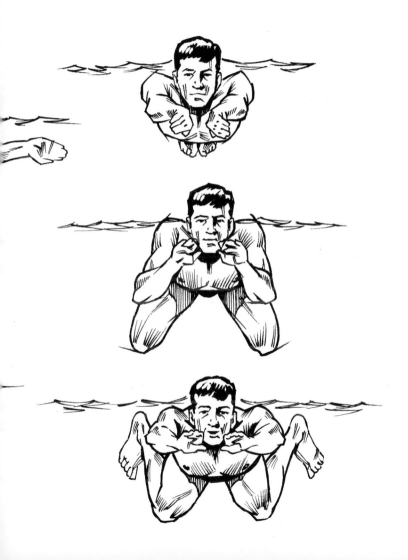

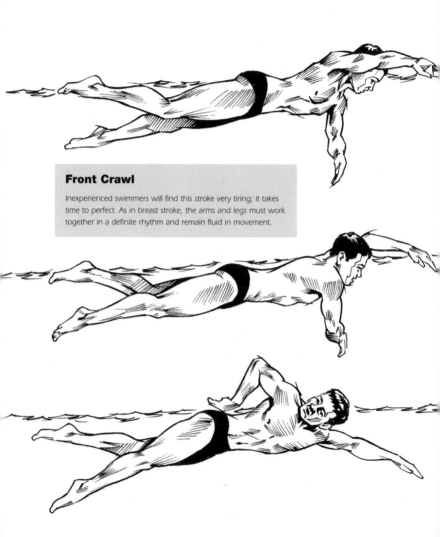

Front Crawl

Inexperienced swimmers will find this stroke very tiring; it takes time to perfect. As in breast stroke, the arms and legs must work together in a definite rhythm and remain fluid in movement.

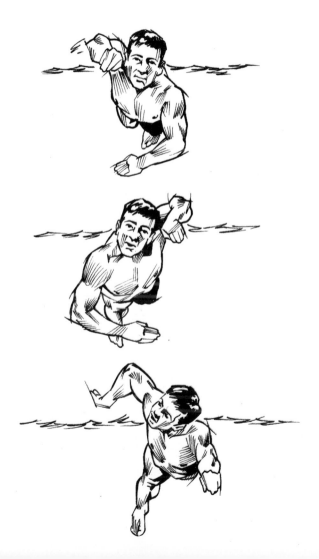

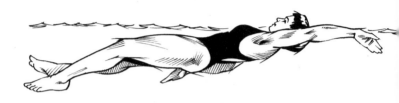

Back Stroke

The arm stroke begins with the little finger entering the water first. The arm is then pulled back until the fingers brush the thigh. The legs beat up and down in a similar action to the front crawl.

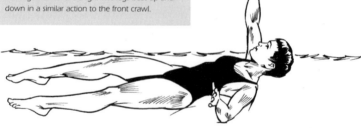

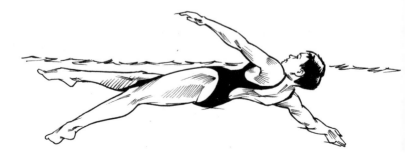

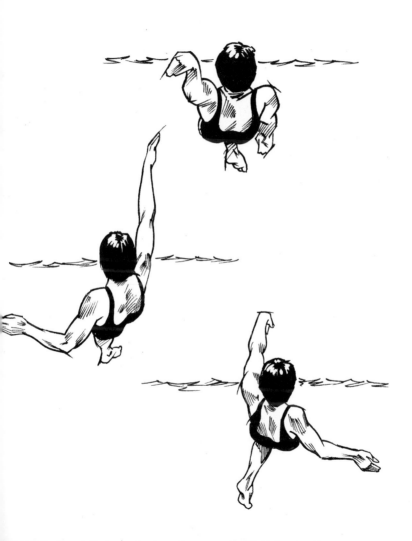

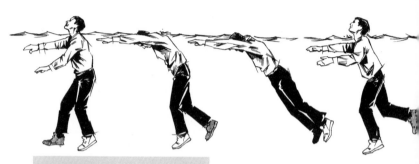

Staying Afloat

- Float upright and take a deep breath.
- Lower your face into the water and bring your arms forward to rest at water level. Relax until you need more air.
- Raise your head above the surface, tread water, exhale then take another breath.

H.E.L.P.

The Heat Escape Lessening Posture (with buoyancy aid):

- Curl up your body as much as possible.
- Try and hug your knees as close to your body as you can.
- Keep your body movements to an absolute minimum to prevent the expenditure of energy.

Timed Swim

Note the time it takes to swim one length of the pool as fast as you can. Most pools are 25 m (82 ft) long and should take between 40-45 seconds. Now try the following routine:

1 Swim four lengths in three minutes
2 Take three minutes rest
3 Swim eight lengths in six minutes
4 Take six minutes rest
5 Swim sixteen lengths in twelve minutes
6 Take six minutes rest
7 Swim eight lengths in six minutes
8 Take three minutes rest
9 Finally, swim four lengths in three minutes

Endurance Swim

Swim for one hour at an easy pace, changing strokes as required. Record how far you swam. Next time, try to increase your distance by three laps.

Drown-Proofing

Drown-proofing is about staying afloat and alive in the water. Lay face down in the water with arms and legs fully extended like a star. Push down with the arms to raise the head and take a breath of air. Hold your breath and relax again. You will float just below the surface even when wearing heavy clothing and boots. Blow the air out gently until you need a breath again and once again push down with arms and raise the head.

Just how long you can survive using this technique depends on water temperature. The colder the water, the sooner the onset of hypothermia. Salt water is more buoyant than fresh water and helps us keep afloat, but we must not swallow it. Ingesting salt water will not only lead to nausea and vomiting but also to dangerous dehydration.

H.E.L.P.

The Heat Escape Lessening Posture (H.E.L.P.) is a position where you curl up in the water to conserve as much body heat as possible. Hypothermia or the critical loss of body heat undoubtedly plays a role in many of the drownings in British waters. To achieve the H.E.L.P. position, a life jacket or some other buoyancy aid is required.

CHAPTER SEVEN

Cycling

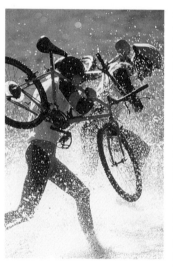

Cycling is an excellent exercise and a good alternative to running. If running aggravates old knee injuries, cycle instead. On a bicycle, you can cover more miles and so you are guaranteed a change of scenery. The only disadvantage of cycling is the ever-present risk of a traffic accident. Unfortunately, the cyclist's own good sense and skill is not enough to protect him, as his safety often lies with other road users. In addition, a collision between a car and a cyclist is a very one-sided affair, no matter who is at fault. Consequently, a lot of extra care has to be taken if you decide that cycling is for you.

A bicycle requires a reasonably large financial outlay. If you are going to include cycling in your training programme, you will need a good quality racing bike. Avoid mountain bikes. Although it is fun to ride along the rough cross-country tracks, the inevitable spills can result in injuries that will set back your training programme.

Clothing

A hard safety helmet is essential when cycling. Every year, many cyclists are killed or seriously hurt as a result of head injuries. Cycling shoes are also very important. They come in two types. One design snaps on to the pedals, while the other is secured by toe-clips. Invest in a pair of cycling shorts. These are padded in all the right places and will save the cyclist a lot of unnecessary discomfort.

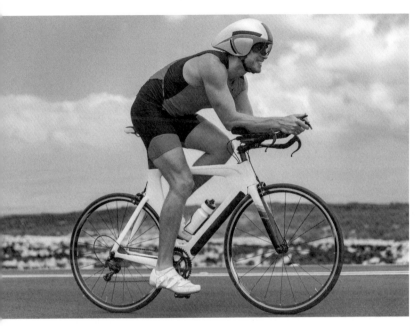

Water bottles are another must for the long-distance cyclist. Two one-litre ($1\frac{3}{4}$ pint) bottles are a good idea, one filled with water and the other with an isotonic drink. The drink will replace all the lost energy without disturbing your blood chemistry, and the water can be poured over your head to refresh your tired body!

Cycling gloves are another excellent buy. These will reduce the blisters that form on the palms as a result of the continual pressure, which is most severe when you are climbing hills.

Wear a cyclist's mask if you intend to ride through heavy traffic. These are constructed from neoprene rubber and fitted with a charcoal filter. They do tend to restrict breathing when you are working hard, but they will prevent sore throats and filter out much of the noxious fumes

Essential items of kit for cycling include a hard safety-helmet, a pair of cycling shorts for maximum comfort and protection, as well as a pair of special cycling shoes.

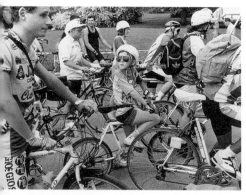

You can get in some useful and at the same time highly enjoyable cycle training with the whole family at a fun event, such as the one pictured here at Crystal Palace.

from vehicle exhausts. Sunglasses offer some protection from flying grit and the multitude of insects which fill the air in the summer.

The cyclist's vest is another useful piece of kit. The many pockets around the back can be used to carry a lot of essential equipment. On the subject of equipment, always carry a tyre pump, two spare inner tubes and a puncture repair kit.

Additional Equipment

Training all year will mean that you will sometimes ride at night. Make sure that you have bright, dependable lights. These should comprise a red rear light and reflectors and a good front light. Consider fitting a strobe light on the front. These are easily seen by other road-users and well worth the extra money. A reflective band, worn across the shoulder, is another good safety item. You cannot be too safe!

You will not need many clothes during a heavy training session. During cold weather, wear a long-sleeved vest and tracksuit trousers. Avoid water-proofs when training since even fabrics that can 'breathe' trap some condensation. Select clothing with bright colours so that they will be highly visible to other road users. Avoid black and dark colours.

Riding Tips

Adjust the saddle as high as possible without it becoming uncomfortable. This will relieve some strain on the back and legs. Although cycling mainly works the legs, the arms and back also have to cope with a lot of strain, particularly when climbing hills. Try to keep the ankles as low as possible when peddling, since this will reduce the strain on the calf muscles.

Select the right gear for the road and try to maintain an even pace. Force the pace on hills to give yourself a good work-out. A rest can be snatched on the downhill section.

A cyclist has the same rights and responsibilities as any other vehicle.

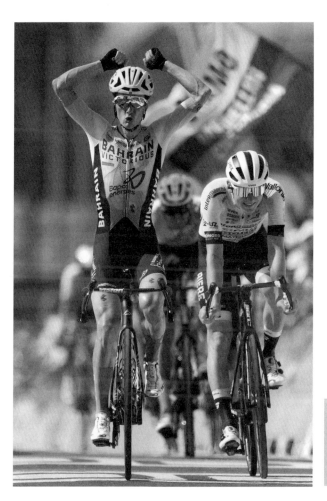

Look no further than the Tour de France for inspiration for your cycling training. The competitors are superb athletes at the absolute peak of fitness. Try to follow their example!

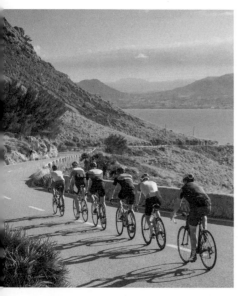

Stay at least 1 m (3 ft) from the kerb; this allows you room to avoid parked cars – and car doors opening! When turning or overtaking stationary vehicles, look behind you and then give the correct signal so that your intentions are clear to other road users.

Keep a sharp eye on the road ahead for obstacles such as pot-holes, debris and glass from traffic accidents, but never swerve out suddenly. If faced with a pot-hole or some other obstacle, brake, check behind you and then go around it.

When turning right, always check behind you before pulling out onto the crown of the road. In heavy traffic, try and keep up with the flow, but be careful when travelling up the inside of a slower vehicle. Keep alert for traffic pulling in front of you at junctions. On wet roads, keep your brakes on slightly to ensure that you can stop in an emergency. Avoid the white lines and lane markers since these become

Head for the open road! But always remember to take an emergency repair kit with you, plus an isotonic drink and chocolate or other high-energy snacks.

treacherous when wet. Take it easy until you get the feel of the bike and the local roads. Buttocks have to take a lot of abuse and this will be a major source of discomfort, initially. This problem tends to diminish as your riding technique improves and you learn to place less weight on the saddle. Keep in as low a gear as possible. This ensures that the legs are always working against the maximum resistance. Change to a higher gear when climbing hills and remain in the saddle as long as possible. On very steep climbs, you may have to use your body weight by standing on the pedals, but modern bike gears with their wide range tend to make this unnecessary.

Reschedule your cycling if the conditions are wet or windy. Poor weather takes all the pleasure out of the training and only adds to the danger. High, gusty winds are the worst hazards; they can blow you across the road. Braking in the wet also has its problems. Apply both brakes together.

Training

Stage One: Cycle for ten minutes to get the leg muscles warmed up and then time yourself over a 16-km (10-mile) circuit. This should be completed in around 40 minutes. Cool down as you cycle home.

Stage Two: This involves a 32-km (20-mile) circuit which, at a fast pace, should be completed in around 85 minutes. Select a route with plenty of hills and the minimum of traffic.

Stage Three: This is a 80-km (50-mile) circuit with some hilly sections. Maintain a good even pace and aim to complete the course in approximately four hours. Take liquids frequently and snacks when required. Choose a long, straight, level piece of road to eat and drink on the move.

Bike Maintenance

With cycling, the work does not end with the session. The bike still has to be maintained and kept in good working order. Clean and dry the bike. Lubricate all the bearings, chains and cables. Check and adjust the brakes, replacing brake cables when necessary. Check that the wheel bearings are in good condition and that the tyres are inflated to the correct pressures. Pay particular attention to the gear-changing mechanism, making sure that it is free from grit. Stow the bike away safely.

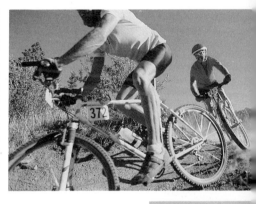

Injuries

A sore backside is very unpleasant. Wash the affected area and dry thoroughly before adding liberal amounts of zinc and castor oil ointment. The most common complaint, however, is sore knees. Knee injuries can be aggravated by a bad riding position. Experiment with different saddle positions. If you are nursing a knee injury, keep the bike in a slightly higher gear. Gravel rash is the most common injury resulting from a fall. Wash the grazed area with mild antiseptic and remove all the dirt.

Note how high the saddle position is here. Do likewise and adjust your saddle as high as possible without being uncomfortable to relieve strain on the back and legs.

CHAPTER EIGHT

Self-Defence

The SAS call it 'close quarter battle' (CQB). To others, it is unarmed combat, self-defence or a useful distillation of the various martial arts. Whatever you choose to call it, this chapter offers a range of techniques that the unarmed civilian can use to counter every form of attack. Self-defence is a basic skill which is part of the training of all elite soldiers. It inspires confidence but requires continual practice. You can never become complacent about your level of skill. The techniques explained here must be practised until they become instinctive. The speed, skill and grace when a particular technique is executed is totally dependent on practice and constant repetition. There are no magic 'death-locks' or two-finger strikes that can easily incapacitate an aggressor. There is, however, a wide range of excellent self-defence techniques which anyone can learn. The secret is training and more training.

The best form of self-defence is to remain inoffensive and 'invisible', while maintaining the bearing and body language which communicate to a would-be attacker that you are no easy target. Many tense situations can be resolved by just walking away. It takes courage – and confidence – to walk away. You cannot fight all the violent idiots in the world, turn your life into a battle-zone and still expect to enjoy a good quality of life. That said, there will always be a situation which proves to be an exception to the rule, a situation where you are faced with physical violence and from which there is no chance of escape or retreat.

The martial arts offer much more than physical self-defence techniques; through years of training, they teach confidence, self-discipline and a whole approach to life.

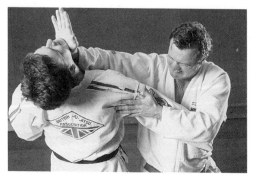

Action and the Law

A famous Japanese karate master once sat down and composed a list of rules for his students. They began with the words: 'There is no first blow in karate'. Today, in most civilised countries of the world, this maxim has been codified into law. Unarmed combat and the martial arts are viewed as weapons capable of deadly force. Unarmed combat should only be used as a last resort. Force must be met with 'reasonable force'.

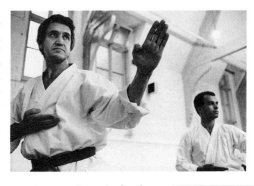

Karate literally translates from the Japanese as 'empty hand'. This popular martial art takes many forms, all characterised by precise, disciplined movements.

The law permits a reasonable response to prevent an attacker from continuing to inflict harm. If you strike the first blow, it can be interpreted as assault with a deadly weapon. You will be required to prove that, had you not acted in self-defence, you were faced with serious injury or worse.

If you ever find yourself in a situation which meets the above criteria, do not threaten your attacker. Explode into action. The resulting encounter should be as fast and furious as it is effective. Many of the techniques in unarmed combat and the martial arts are simple blocks which enable you to counter or deflect the attacker's first strikes. You must be confident that you can do this. This confidence can only come from constant, repetitive training in the self-defence techniques.

Target Areas of the Human Body

These are the areas of the body that we are going to attack; they are called primary targets. Shortly, we will learn how to defend them. Our primary targets are those areas which combatants in boxing or the sporting martial arts are prohibited from striking. A solid strike to these areas should cause immediate incapacitation and immense pain.

Eyes: The eyes are an easy target. From our point of view, they are soft fluid-filled bags of tissue, trapped in narrow funnels of bone. No power is needed to attack the eyes, just a flicked finger will achieve our aims. When the eyes are attacked, the person instinctively looks away and this leaves him open to a range of other strikes. The eyes are very sensitive. A small piece of grit causes great discomfort and may even affect balance. Just a soft blow to the eyes will leave an attacker defenceless and gives you the opportunity to escape from further confrontation.

Nose: Applying any force to the area between the base of the nose and the upper lip can result in severe pain. It can be used as a means of effecting a swift release.

Throat and Neck: The throat and neck are areas where the windpipe, large blood vessels and networks of nerve cells run close to the surface of the body. Consequently, they are very vulnerable to attack. Sharp strikes to the neck and throat areas can disable or kill.

Solar Plexus: The solar plexus is a large soft target which can be attacked using all sorts of strikes. It is important to have strong stomach muscles to protect against blows.

Groin: The groin and genitalia are very sensitive areas in either sex. Attacks to the groin area will disable an attacker. Powerful strikes or kicks to the testicles can kill.

Knee: The knee joint is very delicate and easily crushed or broken by downward thrusting kicks.

There are many other sensitive areas on the human body, but these make smaller, more difficult targets.

On Guard Position

To fight effectively, we must have a stance that enables us to use our maximum speed and power, while providing a good defence against attack. Stand square to the target and slide your favoured foot forward no more than 46 cm (18 in) with the knees slightly bent. Bring up the arms in front of the chest with the elbows tucked in and fingers extended. The leading hand, corresponding to the leading foot, should be held slightly higher than the other.

Moving

Never move out of the guarding position. When moving forward, the front leg leads and the rear leg follows. Movement is smooth and graceful with the feet sliding in a straight line. When moving backwards, the rear leg leads and the front leg follows. The legs are never more than 46 cm (18 in) apart.

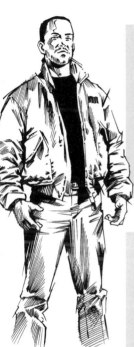

Target Areas of the Body

There are five main vulnerable areas of the body to be targeted in self-defence:

- Eyes. These are highly sensitive; the merest blow wil incapacitate an attacker.
- Nose. Apply force between the base of the nose and upper lip.
- Throat and neck. Extremely vulnerable to attack.
- Solar plexus (stomach area). A large, soft target.
- Groin. The groin and genitalia are very sensitive areas in either sex.
- Knee. The knee joint is quite delicate and can easily be crushed or broken.

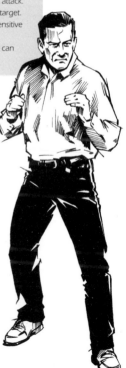

On Guard Position

- Stand square to the target.
- Slide your favoured foot forward 46 cm (18 in) or less, knees slightly bent.
- Place arms in front of the upper chest, elbows tucked in and fingers extending. The leading hand, the same side as the leading leg, should be slightly higher than the other hand.

Never move out of this position in self-defence combat. When moving forward, lead with the front leg and let the rear leg follow. In moving backward, lead with the rear leg and follow with the front. Keep the legs the same distance apart throughout.

Practice

You will need to train with a partner to learn the various techniques. One attacks as the other defends. Always use 'touch contact', with the striking hand or foot just brushing or stopping short of its target. Keep moving and remember to keep your arms up; use the leading hand/arm to block attacks to the head and neck. The rear hand/arm protects the lower half of the body. Keep the chin down to protect the throat. The leading knee bends inwards to protect against a kick or strike to the groin. The centre of gravity is both low and on the centre-line of the body. Weight should be equally distributed on both legs. Stay light and move on the balls of your feet. Parry straight punches and move inside wide, sweeping ('round-house') punches. Do not try to duck or lean back from a punch; if you get the timing wrong you could take the full force of the blow.

Blocking

Practice with your sparring partner trying to touch your forehead with a straight-arm technique. If he attacks with his left hand, use your right arm to block or deflect the blow. If he attacks with his right hand, use your left hand/arm to block the technique. The difference between deflecting and blocking is simple. A block uses brute force to counter the blow. A good block can break your attacker's wrist or arm. In contrast, a punch is deflected by using the attacker's own momentum to sweep the attacking arm further in the direction in which it is travelling. A round-house punch, for example, would be deflected back across the attacker's body, throwing him off balance and exposing his back and the attacking side of his body.

There are other ways of dealing with curving round-house techniques. Have your sparring partner throw a round-house punch. As the attack develops, step forward and to the side, to place yourself inside your opponent's technique. Alternatively, you can either move away from the technique or use your forearm to block his arm.

The guarding position will soon become second nature. Most right-handers will lead with the left leg and hand, keeping the right hand and leg coiled back to launch powerful strikes. Remember, while you are still novices, your techniques should be slow. The attacker should strive not for speed but for technical perfection while giving his or her opponent the opportunity to practice good technical blocks.

Finger Strike

From the guard position, practice shooting the leading hand with two fingers spaced to attack your opponent's eyes. Speed, not power, is important in this technique. It is a very fast technique that is very difficult to counter. Relax the body. Tightly knotted muscles make for slow, unco-ordinated movements. Shift the weight to the leading foot and lunge forward. Go for both eyes, keeping all the fingers open. Do not make the classical two-finger strike since this will alert the attacker. Because it is hard to counter simple strikes like this one, you can start to see the importance of keeping strangers out of your personal space.

Many of the techniques used in the martial arts consist of simple but highly effective blocks which allow you to counter or block even the most powerful blow.

Edged Palm

The side of the open hand is a good weapon and ideal for attacking the neck and the groin area. If grabbed from behind, a swinging, back-handed strike with the edge of the palm to the attacker's groin will force anyone to let go and reconsider their intentions.

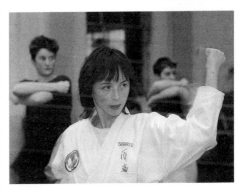

Palm Strike

If you were asked to punch a brick wall as hard as possible, you would be foolish if you did not hold back and execute a very controlled punch. But if you were asked to strike the same wall with your open palm, you could probably deliver the technique with a lot more energy and power.

We start all of our attacks with our hands open. This communicates a lack of obvious aggression. Hands left open and held high to guard your own body gives the thug a false sense of security. This false security will ensure your attacker leaves him or herself open for a fast counter-attack. The palm strike is formed by opening the fingers and flexing the wrist so that the hand is at 90 degrees to the wrist. The strike is delivered to the attacker's chin using the power of the arms and shoulders combined with a fast twist of the hips.

The twisting motion starts from the waist and the strike is unleashed at the last moment when it has the full weight of the body behind it. Do not draw the palm back before you start to move into the strike since this will telegraph your intentions to your attacker. Practice this technique with your sparring partner but remember to only use touch contact. This control is the hallmark of the accomplished empty-handed fighter. In addition, you should be working with a pad or bag to develop speed and power. Ask your sparring partner to hold the training bag at shoulder level.

The base of the bag now provides you with a target at head height. Strike this with five repetitions of fast, hard strikes. The rear hand will always deliver the hardest technique since it can be executed with a hip twist. Start in the guard position. As you shuffle quickly into the attack, flex the attacking shoulder and hips behind you, keeping the weight on the rear leg. The shoulders and hips then uncoil as the hand moves forward to deliver a powerful strike with the palm.

Practice with both the leading and the rear hands. Do five fast repetitions with both techniques. Less power is developed with a leading hand strike but it has the advantages of speed and surprise.

REMEMBER: Drop back in to your guard position between strikes. Close the distance to the training bag as quickly as possible with both hands held high and open. Speak to your 'attacker' in a pleading voice, "No, please don't run away."

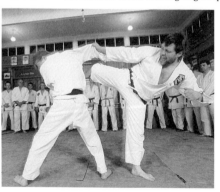

This ju-jitsu move illustrates the effectiveness of the hip-twist and coiling of the leg in the delivery of a powerful leg strike (see pages 121–122 for instructions on kicks).

Elbow Strike

This strike, with all the body's energy and power focused onto the small surface area of the elbow, can be devastating. The elbow strike is fast and powerful; it combines both force and the element of surprise. Face your opponent with arms held high and hands open in a pleading attitude. Keeping your hand high, quickly move the elbow of the leading arm towards the side of your attacker's jaw. Twist the shoulders and hips to deliver the strike with maximum force. Stepping into the target delivers even more force. Practice this technique with your partner holding the training bag. Train with the leading arm first, since it delivers more power with this technique. Step into the bag, roll the hips and shoulders and snap out the strike. Your sparring partner will certainly be able to tell you about the power of this technique. Delivered correctly, it should knock him backwards. Do five repetitions with both arms.

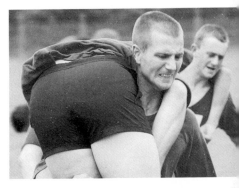

It is useful in self-defence or CQB training to become accustomed to handling other people and their body mass. Practise this 'fireman's lift' with a partner.

The Head Butt

An aggressive move, not recommended for self-defence. To avoid becoming the victim of a head butt, the guard position will ensure you stay at arm's length.

Knee Strike

A knee strike delivered to your attacker's groin will disable him. From the guard position, keep the hands high and open. Shift the weight to the front leg and sink down, before driving the rear knee into the groin area. You can then grab your attacker and deliver another fast strike with the front knee. Other targets for this strike include the solar plexus and the outside of the thigh. Thigh strikes will collapse your attacker's leg. Deliver a short, sharp strike to the outside of his thigh and move away.

Kicks

Do not deliver a front kick with the ball of the foot. This is easy for the attacker to spot and block. Rather, turn to one side and coil the leg before striking with the side of the foot. The kick should be delivered with hip-twist and the target areas for this kick are the shins, knees, thighs or solar plexus.

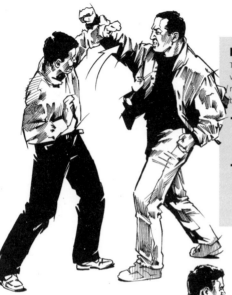

Blocking a Blow

The blocking movement is a sure-fire way of countering any straight arm or round-house (swinging) punch with basic brute force.

- If your assailant or sparring partner attacks with his or her left hand, use your right arm to block or counter the blow.
- Alternatively, if he or she attacks with the right hand, use your left arm to block the blow.

Kick

To deliver a really powerful strike:

- Turn to one side and coil the leg.
- Make your strike with the leg fully extended.
- Make contact with your opponent's body with the side of the foot while twisting the hips.
- Aim for the shins, knees, thighs or solar plexus.

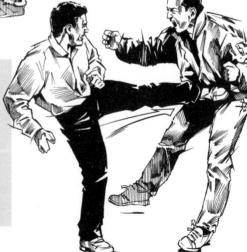

Combination Strikes

Now that we have learnt some basic techniques, we have to learn to string them together. The individual techniques are like words in a language; combinations teach you to speak in simple sentences. As always, we start from the guard position with the left leg forward (for right-handed people). Left-handers should lead with their right leg. Strike with a straight left finger strike to your 'attacker's eyes'. The first technique serves as a 'ranging shot' and starts to close the distance between you and your assailant. Always aim for the eyes because, even if you miss, it will serve to distract your opponent. Because you have started from a stance with the left leg and shoulder forward, a right palm strike is ready to fly.

Rotate the hips and drive your palm into your assailant's chin. This action should rotate your own body to the left, automatically 'cocking' any left-handed technique. Unwind from the hips and drive your left elbow into your attacker's chin or nose. For good measure, snap up your right knee to the groin area to finish the combination. Practice getting these four strikes into a rhythm. Each strike coils the body, 'cocking' the action on the next strike. The movements should flow one into the other without conscious thought.

Use your legs to alter the distance between you and your target. Your leg techniques should be the most powerful. Always 'strike through' the target, aiming for a spot below or behind the target area and thereby generating the maximum power. I guarantee that this combination will disable the biggest of attackers, even when used by a woman of slight build. The secret is practice to perfect the techniques.

SAS-Style Training

The SAS believes in the five-second fight. A fight lasting longer than five seconds promises to have no winners. To fight effectively for five seconds takes months of training. Learn all the techniques and train with a partner. Take it easy and practice your techniques slowly at first. Think carefully about your stance and timing. Alternate the roles of attacker and defender with your sparring partner and get into the habit of constructively criticising each other's techniques. Constant repetitions are the answer to building speed. Perform five repetitions of techniques and combinations of techniques as quickly as possible.

Remember that balance and the quick transfer of body weight from one leg to the other are the secrets of speed.

Breathing

Correct breathing is very important in self-defence and the martial arts. The following exercise will help you develop the right breathing rhythm. Stand relaxed, with feet one shoulder width apart, hands on hips and leaning forward very slightly. Raise your chest and focus on a point 2.5 cm (1 in) above your navel. Breathe in through your nose to the count of 'five'. Hold your breath for the count of 'five'. Expel the air forcibly through your mouth to the count of 'five'. This tidal breathing has been shown to help overcome anxiety and focus the mind. Finish any training period with this simple breathing exercise.

Breathing is also very important when delivering a strike. Just as the blow lands on the target, violently expel the air in your lungs. At the same time, tighten your stomach muscles to help protect the solar plexus in the event of a counter-strike to that area.

Special Exercises

For hand speed and strength, stand with the right or left hand open in front of you. To the count of ten, open and close the hand as quickly as possible. On 'ten', make as tight a fist as possible and again hold for the count of ten. Build up to 100 repetitions of this exercise. Your hands and arms will soon start to ache but you will develop speed and power. After the exercise, relax the hands and arms and shake them around to loosen them up.

CQB One

1 Warm up

2 Stretching exercises

3 Fitness Programme Three (see page 42). In between sets of the fitness programme, introduce three lines of shuttle runs with each line approximately 15 m (49 ft) apart. Sprint to the end of the first line and deliver ten finger strikes. Sprint to the second line and perform ten palm strikes. Sprint to the end of the third line and execute ten elbow strikes. Sprint to the end of the first line and deliver ten knee strikes.

Use a three-minute recovery period to do some deep breathing.

CQB Two

Use this exercise regime for endurance and co-ordination. Skip for three minutes. Punch the speed-ball for three minutes. Work with the training bag for three minutes.

Skipping is an excellent exercise and requires co-ordination. Persevere with this exercise since it is well worth the effort. Use a heavy rope and stay on the balls of your feet. As you become practised, speed up, occasionally doing a double beat and a crossover.

The speed-ball takes a long time to really master. Apart from stamina, it requires timing and good hand-eye co-ordination. Start by lightly punching the bag, hitting it on the second or third rebound with alternate hands. Only practice makes perfect.

Three minutes of solid punching will release all your pent-up frustrations. Get your sparring partner to hold the bag while you strike it. Practice your combinations. Lead with a straight left and then cross with a right hook. Move around the bag for the full three minutes. Do three sets of exercises with three minute's recovery time in between each set.

Yoga and Flexibility

A yoga course is probably one of the best ways of working towards total flexibility. By holding some of these seemingly impossible postures, the muscles actually relax and ligaments are stretched. Like everything else in life, yoga requires a lot of hard work, but once increased flexibility has been gained, it is easily maintained.

The many and various positions help to relieve the stiffness and pain acquired through more vigorous forms of exercise. Yoga also helps to soothe the mind and relieve stress and tension.

Self-Discipline

Discipline in the SAS is self-discipline. No one tells you to shave, wash your clothes or to get a haircut. This is simply expected of you. You have to think for yourself. Self-discipline is the hardest form of discipline and it appears to be beyond the reach of many people. They need someone constantly to organise them and tell them what they must and must not do. Always strive to improve your weaknesses and inadequacies. Self-discipline is the first step to achieving this. With self-discipline comes the ability to control your techniques and your temper.

CHAPTER NINE

Injuries

We are going to be training hard and so it is very important that we learn to distinguish between the sort of injuries that will heal themselves with rest and those that require medical supervision.

The SAS training programme will often take us to the limits of our endurance and so it is also important that we learn to recognise and deal with acute medical problems such as hypothermia, hyperthermia and exhaustion. Of course, the risk of incurring any of these problems can be minimised. We should always warm up and warm down before and after exercise. We should push ourselves towards our physical and mental limits only by gradually building on the exercises.

Accidents and injuries often occur when we ignore the 'danger signals' of extreme fatigue. Every fit man and woman can successfully complete the exercises in this book but you must move at your own pace. Set your own personal standards for runs, exercises, weights and endurance work.

Feet and Legs

We are going to be putting a lot of stress on our feet and legs during this training programme so, in our short tour of common injuries, the lower limbs are a good place to start. First, let us start with the advice that sports doctors give to teams of professional runners:

- ◆ Most foot injuries can be avoided by extensive warming-up exercises and purchasing good running shoes.
- ◆ Good sports shops measure the width and length of their client's feet to ensure that they purchase close-fitting running shoes.
- ◆ The sole of the shoe should be flexible and the heel cushioned.
- ◆ Running shoes should fit snugly and the heel design should prevent the ankle from moving from side to side.
- ◆ There should be about 1 cm ($\frac{1}{2}$in) clearance between the big toe and the front of the shoe with no rough edges inside.

Twisted Ankle: This is the most common type of injury in both sports and everyday life. It has been estimated that every day some 5,000 people go to their local doctor or casualty department with 'twisted ankle'. What has happened is that a sharp, sideways twist of the ankle has stretched, or torn, one or more of the small ligaments which connect the bones of the lower leg to the bones of the upper foot. The ankle is often very swollen and tender and there may be bruising around the site of the injury. Your doctor will need to examine the ankle to determine the severity of the injury and may ask for X-rays and special investigations of the joints and tendons to exclude fractures and more serious complications. In most instances, the injuries soon heal and treatment is directed at relieving the pain and swelling. Anti-inflammatory drugs alone may have the younger person back on their feet in only a couple of days.

In contrast, badly torn ligaments or joint injury may require a lower leg plaster cast and rehabilitation exercises. In these cases, further training involving the legs and feet will have to be suspended for up to 10 weeks or possibly longer.

Policeman's Heel: This is a common complaint of runners, especially long-distance runners. It is more common in older people. The major symptom of policeman's heel is a sharp, crippling pain under the heel, which is worse after getting out of bed and placing weight on the foot. Rest can appear to heal the injury but the pain will often return after a long run. What has happened is that the plantar muscles and ligaments, which run underneath the foot from the heel-bone to the toes, have become strained, often because tight calf muscles in the lower leg prevent the ankle from flexing fully.

See your doctor. He or she may recommend physiotherapy or twice-daily exercises to stretch the gastrocnemius muscle and the Achilles tendon. In the interim, much of the pain can be relieved by a course of anti-inflammatory drugs and a Sorborthane heel pad to cushion the heel. In many cases, this complaint can be avoided by ensuring that the leg muscles are fully exercised and stretched during the warm-up period.

If the symptoms persist, injections of steroids or a local anaesthetic underneath the heel usually cure this condition.

Stress Fractures: These occur most frequently in the calcaneus or heel bone. The ankle may be swollen and there is quite severe pain on walking. Although easily detected by X-ray, medical advice as to the treatment often varies. Some doctors recommend iced water to reduce the swelling, followed by exercises to flex the ankle. Later, when the swelling is reduced, the patient is advised to walk as long and as far as the pain permits.

Small stress fractures result from the pounding we give our feet when running on hard surfaces. Consequently, we can reduce the risk of this quite serious injury by choosing well-fitting running shoes with heavily cushioned soles and by avoiding running on roads and other hard surfaces.

The most extreme form of this injury is seen in parachutists who have suffered a bad landing, but it can also result from jumping on to a hard surface and landing on the heel. In these cases, the heel bone can be completely broken, resulting in three to six months recuperation. It can be avoided by heeding the advice given to all parachutists:

- Before you jump prepare to land with knees and feet together.
- Your knees should be bent such that you can just see your toes.
- Your feet should be horizontal in order to absorb the initial shock of landing across the whole underside of the feet.
- As you hit the ground, much of the shock of landing will be further absorbed by your bent legs.
- The shock is further dissipated by the parachute roll: keeping your knees together and your elbows tucked in close to the body, flex the knees to the side. As you hit the ground, roll, absorbing the now greatly reduced landing shock across your back.

Inflammation of the Joints and Tendons of the Mid Foot: These complaints result from the tendons, ligaments and joints in the feet undergoing a lot of additional strain during intensive training.

Pain is usually experienced only during running or when the affected part is stretched or flexed. Minor injuries are treated with anti-inflammatory drugs. In more severe injuries, the foot is strapped to prevent movement of the inflamed tissue or joint. Most of these injuries will heal quickly.

Runner's Toe: The appearance of 'blood blisters' under the toenails of long distance runners is very common. Unfortunately, this bleeding into the soft tissue underneath the nail often produces a painful swelling. The treatment requires more than a little courage and perhaps should be left to the doctor. The immediate treatment involves puncturing the nail above the blood-blister with a sterile needle. In the long term, the complaint can be prevented by buying more appropriate footwear.

Blisters: Doctors correctly associate blisters with new or badly-fitting shoes. However, blisters are also an inevitable consequence of long-distance walking and running. The immediate treatment simply involves bursting the blister with a sterile needle and covering the affected area with a dry dressing, firmly secured with adhesive plaster. Blisters result from the foot being rubbed by the inside of the shoe or boot. In the short term, the way to prevent this is to grease your feet with baby oil or petroleum jelly and to wear two pairs of socks – all of which helps the feet to move within the shoes with the minimum of friction.

In the long term, the friction which results from continuous exercise will induce a hard, leathery layer of skin on the sides and underside of the feet. There is no way to accelerate this process. Bathing the feet in chemicals such as methylated spirits does produce a thin, horny layer of skin but it is quickly sloughed off.

Inflammation of the Achilles Tendon: This is a common complaint in those playing football, volley ball or tennis and in sprinters, middle and long- distance runners and even ballet dancers. Usually, only the sheath surrounding the Achilles tendon is affected, but in more severe cases the tendon itself becomes inflamed. This is a very painful condition. The affected individual becomes aware of mild pain in the back of the leg during exercise and this may disappear only to become much more severe after training. In the morning, the affected individual experiences stiffness and pain which gradually disappears during the day.

Achilles tendonitis is the crippling complaint suffered by soldiers wearing high combat boots. Shoes which hold the feet in such a way as to shorten the Achilles tendon can also cause this condition. It has also been associated with intensive running up hills, rigid training shoes and training on hard surfaces. People with abnormally tight hamstrings or gastrocnemius muscles are also predisposed to inflammation of the Achilles tendon. The simple treatment of this condition consists of oral anti-inflammatory medication and ice-baths.

Medical investigations will generally try to identify the cause by examining the leg muscles and by looking at the patient's gait – an abnormal gait is often apparent from the unusual pattern of wear on the patient's training shoes. Some unfortunate patients will need surgery. The patient's normal training programme is suspended throughout the course of the investigations and treatment in favour of regular sessions of cycling and swimming. Only about half of the patients with this condition will be able to return to full training; the rest are able to train less intensively and may be troubled by occasional recurrences of pain. A very few will be unable to resume physical training or sports.

Rupture of the Achilles Tendon: This condition rarely occurs in healthy tendons. In some people, the part of the tendon closest to the heel is not well supplied with blood vessels and it begins to degenerate. The weakened tissue then breaks as a result of undue strain on the tendon or a sudden contraction of the calf muscles.

Perhaps not surprisingly, this injury tends to be associated with sports such as badminton, squash and the martial arts. As the tendon severs, the individual often hears a cracking sound or claims that he was hit or kicked behind the heel. There is often very little pain and no difficulty in walking and the person concerned believes that they have only experienced some minor injury. It is only two hours later, as swelling and bruising develops on the leg immediately above the heel, that the person becomes aware of the injury. If the patient intends returning to full activity, this condition must be treated as a medical emergency. The sooner it is diagnosed, the easier it is to treat. It may be possible to treat those cases identified within the first 48 hours by plaster cast immobilisation (eight weeks). Other patients face surgical repair and plaster cast immobilisation for six weeks.

Shoulders and Upper Limbs

Dislocated Shoulder: Displacement of the upper bone of the arm (the humerus) from the shoulder joint often results from a fall on an outstretched hand. This is an anterior dislocation. The other type of dislocation, posterior dislocation, is rarely seen as a sporting injury, although it can result from a fall onto the elbow.

A dislocated shoulder is easy to diagnose. The patient finds that the least painful position involves supporting the affected arm across his or her chest. The normal curvature of the shoulder is lost and there may be a very obvious hollow underneath the deltoid muscle. Under general anaesthetic, the humerus can be pulled and rotated back into position. The arm is then supported by a sling, which prevents rotation or abduction of the shoulder joint, for two to three weeks. At three weeks, the patient is encouraged to undertake increasingly demanding exercises to increase joint mobility, but a return to full training may be delayed for another two to three months.

Tendonitis of the Shoulder: This can start as an extreme and sudden pain in the shoulder which may become worse on movement. The condition results from inflammation of the tendons within the shoulder, usually from the movements involved during intensive training. If left untreated, the inflammation may result in deposition of calcium and some restriction of movement. This condition responds well to injections of anti-inflammatory drugs, such as corticosteroids, and local anaesthetic to ease the worst of the pain. The healing process may also be helped by immobilising the patient's arm in a sling. During the period of rehabilitation, isometric exercises and free isotonic exercises with weights are recommended. These exercises strengthen the affected muscles and tendons.

Frozen Shoulder: This is a very poorly understood condition. It results in quite severe pain which is often worse at night. Remedial exercises and steroid injections play a role in treatment but the most important factor is time because, although the symptoms may persist for a year or more, the condition is self-limiting and the shoulder will eventually return to normal.

Tricipital Tendonitis: This causes quite severe pain when the elbow is flexed or rotated. Once again, the condition can result from over-use of the tendons and muscles associated with the elbow. Patients will be advised to rest, while anti-inflammatory drugs and light exercises will restore the elbow to its normal state.

Tennis Elbow: This very common complaint is characterised by soreness over the inner bony protuberance of the elbow (lateral epicondyle of the humerus). This is the point of insertion of the ulnar extensor muscle of the wrist which is very important in wrist extension. Continual flexing of the wrist, as occurs in racquet games, may result in inflammation of the muscle and tendon where it attaches to the humerus. The condition responds well to rest, steroid injections and local anaesthetic injections to ease the soreness in the elbow.

Golfer's Elbow: This results from stress placed on ligaments in the area of the outer bony protuberance of the elbow or the medial epicondyle. The strain occurs during wrist-flexing in golf and weight-lifting (particularly snatch lifts). The tenderness, which is localised in the area of the medial epicondyle, quickly responds to rest and anti-inflammatory drugs. In severe cases, injections of local anaesthetic are used to control the pain.

Frictional Tenosynovitis of the Wrist and Hand: This also results from unusual stress being placed on the wrist during sports or exercises. The pain is localised at the back of the wrist and thumb, and results from inflammation of the sheaths of the extensor tendons of the wrist.

The affected hand is usually splinted for seven to ten days, to minimise movement of the tendons within the inflamed sheath. Splinting combined with a short course of anti-inflammatory drugs usually results in a cure.

Medical Emergencies

In most sports and activities, the risk of serious injury and unconsciousness is confined to rare and unusual accidents. However, in the martial arts and in 'risk activities' such as parachuting, rock climbing, hill-walking and canoeing, to mention just a few, the risk is more immediate. Once a serious accident has occurred, the immediate care which can be provided by anyone with a little knowledge may make a huge difference to the outcome. That care is covered by the simple mnemonic, ABC. But first, the rescuer should perform several other vital tasks:

- Check that the path to the casualty is safe. If it is not, take the necessary steps to ensure that you can reach the casualty safely.
- Make sure that someone else contacts the emergency services. You can only provide immediate aid.
- Ask a third person to make short, simple notes on when and how the accident happened. These notes will be invaluable for the medical staff at the hospital, who will otherwise have to use their imaginations.
  Move to the casualty and ascertain his or her level of consciousness.
  Is he/she alert and obviously breathing?
  Does he/she respond to your voice?
  Does he/she respond to pain?
  Is the casualty totally unresponsive?

A is for Airway: If the casualty is unresponsive or only partly responsive, check that their airway is clear. Open the casualty's mouth and use two fingers to check for obstructions such as blood, vomit and broken teeth in the mouth and throat. Clear these obstructions.

B is for Breathing: Place your face close to the casualty's body and see if his or her chest is rising and falling. Put your hand close to the casualty's mouth and nose and feel for the exhalation of air. Listen for sounds of breathing or obstruction.

C is for Circulation: Check the carotid pulse on the side of the casualty's neck to ensure that his/her heart is still beating. If the casualty is not breathing, or if his/her heart has stopped beating, Cardiac-Pulmonary Resuscitation (CPR) must be started immediately. This is not the place to teach CPR, which is a very practical skill complicated by special considerations in, say, cases of drowning or possible spinal injury. CPR should be taught by your local St John's Ambulance instructor or by first-aid instructors in your sports club or gym. As part of the instruction, you will be taught how to stabilise the casualty and place them in a recovery position.

Hypothermia

This life-threatening condition is usually associated in people's minds with severe winter conditions on the mountains. In fact, there are different types of hypothermia and it is possible to become hypothermic on a reasonably hot day. In hypothermia, the body's core temperature, the temperature deep within the body, undergoes a dangerous decline. All of the bodily functions associated with life are dependent on a stable core temperature of around 37°C (98.9°F). Hypothermia is classified into three main types:

Rapid or 'Immersion' Hypothermia: The affected individual's core body temperature is reduced by severe cold stress, as happens when a person falls into very cold water. Because it is the environment which is reducing the core

Body Temperature	Symptoms
37°C (98.6°F)	The person's pace begins to slow. He or she may keep stumbling and complain of muscle cramps.
35°C (95°F)	Intense shivering which stops as the condition worsens.
33-32°C (91.4-89.6°F)	Confusion and amnesia.
30°C (86°F)	Progressive loss of consciousness.
29°C (84.2°F)	Progressive decline in pulse rate and breathing.
27°C (80.6°F)	Loss of tendon and skin reflexes.
24-20°C (75.2-68°F)	Build-up of fluid in lungs; heart stops.

temperature, these casualties can still produce body heat and usually respond well to treatment.

'Exhaustion' Hypothermia: This is seen in marathon runners and may have been responsible for at least one death on SAS Selection. The person runs out of energy and is unable to maintain his or her body core temperature, even though the ambient temperature may not be cold. These casualties are more difficult to treat. An effort must be made to prevent their core temperature falling any further by blocking every possible type of heat loss, because they are no longer producing their own heat. Exhaustion hypothermia may be complicated by blood and body fluids being shunted into the tissues, thus decreasing blood pressure and blood circulation.

Slow Hypothermia: This often occurs in elderly people after an accident. Losing mobility, their energy levels and consequently their body's core temperature may decline over weeks as they drift into hypothermia.

The treatment of hypothermia can be complicated and is best taught by a qualified first-aider or doctor, not least because the patient can collapse during re-warming. The complications associated with hypothermia, both before and after re-warming, are many and various. The majority are life- threatening. Here I will just outline some general advice.

- Warm, sweet drinks can be administered if the patient is suffering from the first stages of hypothermia and is alert and conscious.
- Allowing the casualty to re-warm spontaneously may save his/her life while doing the least harm. As soon as he/she is discovered, wrap them totally in insulating material – a 'space blanket' or a polythene bag will do. If their outer clothes are wet, quickly change them into dry clothes. Additional warmth can be provided by one of the rescuers sharing a sleeping bag with the casualty. Further protection should be provided from the elements by placing the patient and his companion inside a tent or bivi-bag.
- Treatment of the casualty should always have priority! If the 'rescue party' is sufficiently large, one member can be sent to summon help. Otherwise, wait for help to come. Never leave the casualty alone.
- If the casualty can be carried to habitation, some text-books advise re-warming the patient in a bath of warm water. Do not attempt this unless you have had training in managing hypothermic patients.

Hyperthermia

Heat collapse and hyperthermia are associated with strenuous activity on hot days, marathon and long-distance running and endurance activities. It can also be experienced on cold days if a person has engaged in physical activity wearing full wet-weather kit or an immersion suit. Hyperthermia occurs when the core temperature rises above 37°C (98.6°F). A marathon runner produces 13 times as much heat as he/she would while resting. This might be expected to raise the body's core temperature by 1°C (2.6°F) every eight minutes. It says much about the body's cooling abilities that this does not happen. Well-conditioned athletes can withstand moderate hyperthermia without any ill-effects.

The problem arises when the mechanisms which limit further increases in core temperature fail. The core temperature does not have to rise much above 41-42.5°C (105.8-108.5°F) before the person dies within minutes! The early symptoms of heat stroke resemble those of hypothermia: the pace slows and the person stumbles; he or she may be aggressive and irritable, with a glassy-eyed stare. However, these are also the symptoms of dehydration which, in itself, can also lead to heat stroke since little or no fluid is available to produce sweat. If the person feels unwell or presents with any of the above symptoms, treat as follows:

- Prevent the person from engaging in further exercise.
- Administer water or an isotonic fluid in spaced, moderate amounts.
- Lie the person flat on the ground and elevate his or her legs.
- Sponge the person's body with tepid water (cold water closes down the small blood vessels in the skin and delays further heat loss).
- Seek medical advice. If the casualty suddenly collapses, they will need intravenous fluids and specialist medical support.

Heat stroke, with or without dehydration, is much easier to prevent than treat. The basic rules for avoiding the condition are as follows:

- Wear light, loose clothing during strenuous activity. Even if the weather is cold and wet, the heat produced by your body will keep you warm. Moving across country with a heavy Bergen, most SAS men wear only a windproof smock over their upper body.
- Drink plenty of fluids before and during the activity.
- On hot days, soak your T-shirt and headband in water.

CHAPTER TEN

The Complete Fitness Programme

Now that we have seen the different types of training, it is time for you to decide what you want to achieve. With this fitness programme, the sky is the limit, but you must have a realistic goal for the training you have selected. There is no point doing endurance marches if you want to get fit for competitive rugby.

Assessing Your Own Fitness

When blood is pumped out of the heart, a pressure wave shoots along the arteries at ten times the speed of the blood flow. This is the pulse, and it can be felt anywhere that an artery comes close to the surface. The pulse is an easy way of measuring how fast your heart is beating, and the resting heart beat is an indication of overall cardio-vascular fitness. The pulse can be felt on the wrist (below the thumb), at the temple and on the neck (either side of the windpipe).

Sit down and rest for ten minutes. Measure your pulse rate over the course of one minute. Record the rate for future reference. The resting pulse rate tends to increase with age but, excluding heart and vascular disease, it can be correlated with overall fitness.

Pulse Rate	Fitness
50	very fit
70	fit
80	normal
100	unfit

A much better indication of cardio-vascular fitness is the recovery time or the time it takes your heart to return to a normal rate after exercise. We can assess this with the Step Test.

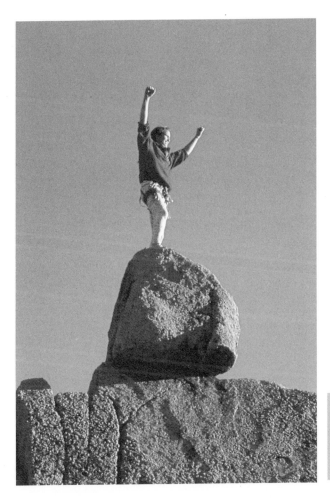

Choose a fitness regime that fits with your lifestyle and into the time you have available, and also offers a realistic goal to give you that great sense of achievement.

Stand in front of a gym bench. Record your resting pulse rate. Start your stop-watch and step up onto the bench and back down onto the floor. Continue this exercise at a regular pace for three minutes. Now, rest for one minute then measure your pulse rate.

Pulse Rate	Fitness
70	excellent
80	good
90	average
100	poor

People over the age of 40 will find that they have a slightly higher resting pulse rate (5-10 beats/min higher than that listed above). Continue checking your pulse and note the time at which it returns to the resting rate. The safe work-out should raise your pulse rate to 140 beats/min.

Selecting the Programme

Your overall level of fitness, the amount of time you wish to spend on any one exercise session and the number of sessions you can manage each week, will help you determine which programme to follow. We start at the lowest level with the Recruit Programme and end with the Professional SAS Programme. In between, we have intermediate and advanced routines.

The Recruit Programme

If you are over-weight, troubled with minor injuries or your overall fitness is low, this is the schedule for you.

WEEK ONE: Aim to exercise for around 40 minutes on alternate days.
Day One: We start with a road walk and run. Jog until you feel uncomfortable and then change to a brisk walk. Open your stride and breathe deeply until your breathing returns to a more moderate rate. When you feel ready, start jogging again. Choose a route or circuit that takes you approximately 40 minutes to complete.
Day Two: This is a rest day, but try some stretching exercises. You may be stiff after your road walk and run, and some gentle stretching will help ease tired muscles.

Day Three: Complete Fitness Programme One (page 37). Do not forget your warm-up, but you can omit the shuttle runs. Programme One is about anaerobic exercises and of course we do not forget those abdominal muscles! Do all the stretching exercises; aim to gain flexibility without straining ligaments and muscles. Try to do five repetitions of every exercise. Take short breaks in between repetitions and three-minute recovery periods between sets of exercises. Do not forget your warm-down exercises. Do them to the best of your ability. Each time you do these exercises, you should notice an improvement. It is worth doing the work-out just to have that shower! You are getting the same enjoyment from the simple pleasures in life as any millionaire. After you have washed, gradually reduce the shower temperature until it is cold. By doing this, in winter the cold air outside the gym will be less of a shock to your system. Wrap up well for the journey home.

Day Four: Although this is a rest day, it gives us a chance to do some more of those abdominal exercises. Do five repetitions of bent knee sit-ups, leg raises, sit-ups and crunches.

Day Five: After warming up and stretching, complete the novice weight training programme on page 70. Work the muscles in the following order: shoulders, chest, back, legs, arms and legs. Because the legs have some of the largest muscles in the body, we exercise them twice. Start with comfortable weights enabling you to carry out the full range of movements.

Day Six: Rest day.

Day Seven: This is the day for our fun swim. Complete as many lengths in 30 minutes as possible. At the end of each length, change to another stroke until you have practised both breast stroke and front crawl. Swimming is a wonderful, relaxing exercise and we have included it at the end of the week to help you recover!

The first week is always the hardest and soon you will find the training much easier. In subsequent weeks, we shall develop our fitness by increasing the tempo of the exercises.

During these three weeks of training, try to eat regular, healthy meals. Also, aim to get to bed early and have a good night's sleep. Try to cut out alcohol and cigarettes.

Week Two	
Day	**Programme**
8	Abdominals – 5 reps in the morning; 5 before retiring.
9	Programme One (page 37).
10	Abdominals – 2 sets.
11	Road walk and run.
12	Abdominals. Increase to 10 reps twice-daily.
13	Novice weights (page 70).
14	Abdominals – twice daily.

Week Three

Day	Programme
15	Run for the full 40 minutes.
16	Abdominals and press-ups. When doing abdominals, do 5 normal press-ups, 5 finger-tip press-ups and 5 wide arm press-ups.
17	Programme One (page 37).
18	Abdominals and press-ups.
19	Novice Weights (page 70).
20	Abdominals and press-ups.
21	Swim.

WEEK FOUR: We are going to train every day and increase our exercise sessions to one hour. Start each morning with ten repetitions of the exercises to work your abdominal muscles. Finish with ten push-ups to exercise the arm muscles! Run on day 22, complete the novice weight training programme on day 23, follow Programme One (page 37) on day 24, then repeat this same pattern of programmes on days 25–27. Pay special attention to your warm-up, stretching and warm-down periods. These should have become second nature by now. After the first month, you can extend the basic programme by making the swimming and runs longer, increasing the number of repetitions and sets for the fitness exercises, and either increasing the weights or number of repetitions for the weight-training exercises. Otherwise, move on to the intermediate programme.

Intermediate Programme

The programme starts every morning when you get out of bed. Spend three minutes on breathing exercises. While you are breathing, focus

Week One

Day	Programme
1	Run 5 km (3 miles). Stretch. Programme Two (page 40).
2	Rest.
3	Intermediate Weights (page 71).
4	Rest.
5	Cycling Stage One. Stretch. Programme Two – increase reps to 10.
6	Rest.
7	Intermediate Weights.

Week Two

Day	Programme
8	Timed swim. Today should be a rest day but a swim will help you unwind.
9	Run 5 km (3 miles). Stretch.
10	Rest.
11	Intermediate Weights.
12	Rest.
13	Cycle. Stretch. Programme Two.
14	Timed swim.

your mind on what you are going to achieve today! Get down on the floor and complete 10 repetitions of each of the following, to be executed in the order given: press-ups, crunchies, finger-tip press-ups, bent knee sit-ups, wide arm press-ups, hand slides, press-ups, leg raises, finger-tip press-ups, sit-ups and wide arm press-ups.

Together with the breathing exercises, these should take no longer than six minutes to complete. The intermediate programme starts with 60-minute sessions, building up to 90-minute sessions by the fourth week.

Week Three	
Day	Programme
15	Programme Two.
16	Rest.
17	Intermediate Weights.
18	Rest.
19	Cycle Stage One. Programme Two.
20	Rest.
21	Intermediate Weights.

Week Four	
Day	Programme
22	Swim.
23	Run. Programme Two.
24	Intermediate Weights.
25	Cycle. Programme Two.
26	Intermediate Weights.
27	Run. Programme Two.
28	Swim.

This demanding training programme and early morning exercises may force you to restructure your social life. But stick with it! I did not say it was going to be easy. Start including complex, carbohydrate-rich foods such as pasta in your daily diet.

Once you have completed the first two weeks of this programme, you should be starting to enjoy the benefits. All the exercises should have become very familiar and you should be able to move from one set of exercises to another without taking rests in-between. However, do take your three-minute rests between sets. Make a note of how long it takes you to complete the whole training session. As your best personal time becomes shorter, maintain the challenge by adding repetitions to each of the exercises and by increasing the training weights.

In the fourth week, we are going to extend each session to 90 minutes and start to work out every day. We will increase the number of sets and make the weight training a little more challenging. Continue with the intermediate programme until you feel ready for the advanced programme.

The Advanced Programme

This is our advanced programme and it really is punishing. I strongly advise all readers to master the intermediate programme first.

Start each day with your breathing exercises, abdominal muscle exercises and push-ups. Do five repetitions of each of the following exercises: crunchies, finger-tip press-ups, bent knee sit-ups, wide arm press-ups, hand slides, normal press-ups, leg raises, sit-ups, finger-tip press-ups and finally more wide arm press-ups. This is one set of exercises. Do three sets in total. The aim is to build stamina. We will have fewer rest days and build up to a climax in the third week when we will complete a 40-km (25-mile) bicycle ride on a hard circuit.

All athletes maintain their fitness by training hard, but the timing of their peak fitness is what really separates the winners from the losers in competitive sports and athletics. The trick is to ensure that you peak on the day of the competition and not in the gym several days earlier. This programme aims to bring you to peak fitness on Day 18 and will help you learn to manage and monitor your own peak fitness.

The next part of the programme will test your recovery times and wet your appetite for further advanced training. On week four, we work every day and we really put in the miles! If, at any time during the training, you feel that you still have energy to spare, add some additional repetitions to the exercises in Programme Three and the weight machine

Week One

Day	Programme
1	Run 8 km (5 miles). Programme 3 (page 42).
2	Rest.
3	Advanced Weights (page 72).
4	Timed Swim Routine (page 107).
5	Cycling Stage Two Advanced Weights – 1 set.
6	Rest.
7	Fast run. Programme Three.

Week Two

Day	Programme
8	Fun swim.
9	Advanced Weights.
10	Rest.
11	Cycling Stage Two. Advanced Weights – 2 reps.
12	Rest.
13	Advanced Weights.
14	Run 8 km (5 miles). Programme Three.

exercises in the advanced weight training programme. Although this programme is very demanding, you should not allow it to take over your life. Your increased fitness should give you more energy and you should take advantage of this to play with your children, spend time with your partner or take up a sport. The trick comes in organising your life so that you make the best use of your spare time and really learn to enjoy it. Also, make sure that you do not become stale and bored with your programme.

Week Three	
Day	Programme
15	Timed swim.
16	Advanced Weights.
17	Rest.
18	Cycling Stage Two.
	Programme Three.
19	Rest.
20	Advanced Weights.
21	Rest.

Week Four	
Day	Programme
22	Programme Three.
23	Run 8 km (5 miles).
24	Advanced Weights.
25	Cycling Stage Two.
26	Programme Three.
27	Advanced Weights.
28	Run 8 km (5 miles).

If you miss a session, work twice as hard on the next one. If you suffer an injury, rest up until you have fully recovered and then continue the programme from where you left off. Your muscles will start to take on more definition and your confidence should also increase. You can be justly proud of what you have achieved!

Split and Double Split Routines

The weight training sessions are staggered to allow you recovery time. It is possible to weight-train every day if we split the body's muscles into three groups and work on one of these each day. (See table opposite.)

When we progress to the professional SAS training programme, we will start to do three sessions every day. It should be possible to weight-train twice a day using double split routines where you train hard for short periods, enabling you to get the most from these intensive sessions.

As you gain more strength and you want to progress further, you can try a schedule of 'super sets'.

Split Routine	
Mon	Shoulders and back.
Tues	Legs.
Wed	Arms and chest.
Thurs	Legs.
Fri	Shoulders and back.
Sat	Arms and chest.

Double Split Routine		
Day	Session 1	Session 2
1	Shoulders/calves.	Back/abdominals.
2	Arms/thighs.	Chest/abdominals.
3	Back/legs.	Shoulders/abdominals.

Maximum Repetitions

At the end of the week, decrease by half the weights in the routines that you are doing and do just one set of exercises with 30 repetitions each. At the end of the fourth week, increase the number of repetitions to 40 and the next week increase them to 50 repetitions. Once you have achieved this, add 2.2 kg (5 lb) to all the weights and drop back to 30 repetitions. In each subsequent week, start adding 10 repetitions to each exercise again.

Super Sets	
Set	Programme
1	15 reps light weight.
2	10 reps 2.2 kg (5 lb) increase.
3	8 reps 2.2 kg (5 lb) increase.
4	6 reps 2.2 kg (5 lb) increase.
5	3 reps maximum.

The Professional SAS Programme

The SAS training programme is tough but only the best get to wear the sand-coloured beret and the winged sword. 'Who dares wins'. Do you dare to win? Do you dare to take on this fitness programme?! We train three times daily, every day. The rationale is to build up stamina without sacrificing strength or speed. Each session is approximately one hour in duration and can be done before work, during the lunch break and in the evening. At weekends, we spend a full day on the hills and swim on Sunday. The rest of Sunday is free time. Although we train with weights every day, we use a split routine.

It is time to monitor your progress and assess what you have achieved. How is the training going? You are now covering a lot of miles and your body should be responding. For variety in your endurance runs,

Weeks One – Four

Day	Session 1	Session 2	Session 3
1	Fun run.	Programme Three plus extra exercises (see page 43).	Advanced Weights (split).
2	Fast run.	CQB 2.	Weights – legs.
3	Endurance run.	Programme Three.	Weights – back, chest.
4	Fun run.	Assault course – 3 laps.	weights – 5 super sets.
5	Cycle endurance.	CQB 2.	Weights – 30 reps.
6	Bergen march – 18 kg (40 lb).		
7	Endurance swim.		
8	Fast run.	CQB 2.	Weights – shoulders, arms.
9	Cycle endurance.	Programme Three.	Weights – legs.
10	Fun run.	Assault course – 5 laps.	Weights – back, chest.
11	Endurance run.	CQB 2.	Weights – 5 super sets.
12	Cycling 24 km (15 miles).	Programme Three.	Weights – 40 reps.
13	Bergen march – 20 kg (45 lb).		
14	Endurance swim.		
15	Fun run	CQB 2.	Weights – shoulders, arms.
16	Fast run.	Programme Three.	Weights – legs.
17	Endurance run.	Assault course.	Weights – back, chest.
18	Fun run.	CQB 2.	Super sets.
19	Cycle endurance.	Programme Three.	Weights – 50 reps.
20	Bergen march – 22 kg (50 lb).		
21	Endurance swim.		
22	Fast run.	CQB 2.	Weights – shoulders, arms.
23	Cycle 24 km (15 miles).	Programme Three.	Weights – legs.
24	Endurance run.	Assault course.	Weights – back, chest.
25	Fun run.	CQB 2.	Super sets.
26	Endurance cycling.	Programme Three.	Weights 30 reps plus 22.2 kg (55 lb).
27	Bergen march – 25 kg (55 lb).		
28	Endurance swim.		

choose different circuits or run the course in the opposite direction on alternate days. Tired muscles? There is nothing like a massage to help aching muscles and help the body relax. Go to a professional masseur or masseuse initially, but you might consider learning this technique, teaching your partner and then asking them to do it. A hot bath is another answer for tired muscles. Add some essential oils. By now, you will know your favourite exercises. We always prefer those things at which we excel. Put more effort into those exercises you hate. You will find some days easier than others; that is the whole idea of this routine. After an endurance exercise we move to a speed session to avoid getting sluggish.

WEEK FIVE: In the fifth week, we change the routine to one session per day as we build up for the Bergen March on day 6. This is equivalent to the SAS endurance march. We start this at 1600 hours on Saturday, carrying 25 kg (55 lb), and march through the night to finish on Sunday.

On Monday, do the advanced weights programme, Tuesday is a rest day, Wednesday: endurance run, Thursday: rest, Friday: cycle endurance, then the march on Saturday. Rest again on Sunday. You should record your best times for the running and cycling sessions. Try to keep to these times in the coming weeks.

WEEK SIX: To prevent ourselves from becoming bored and to keep alive our spirit of adventure, try to spend this week following an outdoor pursuit. Aim to achieve a life-long ambition such as free-fall parachuting, canoeing or rock climbing. Your new-found confidence and strength can be put to the test. Only do light runs and work-outs this week. Leave the weight training alone. This will give you a much needed rest and allow your body to recover and revitalise. Take up a sport or start training for the local half or full marathons. Put your name down for a raft race team.

WEEK SEVEN: On week seven, we return to the hard work of three sessions per day. The break in week six will encourage you to scale new heights and achieve better personal times. Your performance always increases after a rest. The programme is the same as week one but you can add repetitions to the physical training sessions and increase the weights during weight training. Try to improve your times for running and cycling. Add distance to maintain the challenge of the programme!

2 NUTRITION

CHAPTER ELEVEN

Daily Requirements

The body uses food to produce energy, to build, maintain and repair the muscles and other tissues and replace vital chemicals as they are used or lost. Basically, we split 'food' into five major components:

1 Protein
2 Fats
3 Carbohydrates
4 Vitamins
5 Minerals

Amino Acids and Protein

Proteins are long chains of chemicals called amino acids. When we eat meat and nitrogen-rich vegetables, the proteins are broken down into these amino acids in the stomach and intestine. They then pass into the bloodstream where they are ready to be re-synthesised into our own body proteins. Proteins can be composed of as few as 50 amino acids or as many as several hundred amino acids.

There are 25 different amino acids available in our diets. Of these, 15 can be synthesised from other amino acids and these are called the non-essential amino acids. A further ten amino acids cannot be synthesised by our bodies; they must be obtained from the food we eat.

Non-Essential Amino Acids	Essential Amino Acids
Proline	Arginine
Taurine	Histidine
Carnitine	Isoleucine
Tyrosine	Leucine
Glutamine and Glutamic Acid	Lysine
Cysteine and Cystine	Methionine
Glycine	Phenylalanine

Non-Essential Amino Acids	**Essential Amino Acids**
Alanine	Threonine
b-Alanine	Tryptophan
Gamma-Aminobutyric Acid	Valine
Asparagine and Aspartic Acid	
Citrulline	
Ornithine	
Serine	
Glutathione	

The World Health Organisation recommends a daily intake of protein of at least 0.8 grams per kilogram (0.013 oz per lb) of body weight. This would mean that a man or woman weighing about 80 kg (176 lb) needs 64 g (2.3 oz) of protein each day. Athletes and very active people need a lot more.

The British Department of Health recommends that men in the 18–34 age range should consume 1.2 g of protein per kg (0.019 oz per lb) of body weight each day; women in the same age range should eat 1 g of protein per kg (0.016 oz per lb) of body weight. This means that an 80 kg (176 lb) (man needs approximately 96 g (3.3 oz) of protein each day. This could be provided by about 450 g (1 lb) of best steak. Of course, the protein in our diet comes from a much wider range of different types of food than just meat. Proteins are also found in fish, eggs, dairy products and a wide range of vegetables, particularly cereals and legumes such as beans.

The vegetarian therefore faces little difficulty in getting his or her daily requirement of protein and, more particularly, his or her essential amino acids. The vegan faces a more difficult problem and must plan his or her diet much more carefully. The problem faced by the vegan is that protein from any one particular vegetable may be deficient in one or more of the essential amino acids. Fortunately, however, not all plants are deficient in the same essential amino acids. Consequently, in order to meet their daily requirements of the essential amino acids, vegans must eat a large range of vegetables, cereals and green-leaved plants. It is commonly believed that athletes, sportsmen and those undergoing hard physical training benefit from high-protein diets. After all, it is reasoned, these people want to build muscle and muscles are composed of protein. However, doctors are now arguing against the high-protein diet of steak and eggs. We should already obtain sufficient protein and the essential amino acids from a well-balanced diet that contains not only protein but all the other essential components such as sugars, fats, minerals and vitamins. Red meat also contains a lot of saturated fat which is one of the most important factors in heart disease. In addition, fat is a poor energy source for the athlete.

The diet recommended for the professional athlete is rich in complex sugars (carbohydrates) and adequate in protein. High-protein diets are usually poor in energy-producing sugars. This means that the vital supplies of glycogen (the complex sugar in our muscles) are not present to fuel high-intensity training. In addition, excess protein is simply eliminated by the body and this elimination requires extra water. During training, a person on a high-protein diet may become seriously dehydrated.

High-protein diets aside, recent research work has shown that athletes, and those doing heavy physical work or training, may benefit from additional supplements of certain amino acids. These include both essential and non-essential amino acids. They include glycine, aspartic acid/asparagine, arginine, glutamine, serine, taurine, methionine, valine, leucine, isoleucine and cysteine.

Some of these amino acids give rise to other amino acids. For example, methionine is converted to both cysteine and taurine; taurine is important in wound-healing. The essential branched-chain amino acids such as valine, leucine and isoleucine promote muscle growth after intense training. Cysteine, glycine, arginine and glutamine are involved with the maintenance of sugar in the blood. Asparagine/aspartic acid increases endurance in athletes. Your doctor can advise on supplements of these amino acids – some are contra-indicated in certain illnesses – and the recommended dose rate. They are usually supplied in powder form and it is usually recommended that they be taken after a meal. Some are best taken after consuming a high-carbohydrate meal.

At present, the medical advice concerning our daily protein requirements can be summarised as follows:

- High-protein diets are a thing of the past.
- Your diet should include sufficient protein from a wide range of sources including fish, fowl, vegetables, legumes and green-leaved plants.
- Avoid sources of protein which also contain saturated fats (red meat, sausages and hamburgers).

◆ During intensive training programmes, you may benefit from supplements of certain amino acids. If you wish to find out more about these supplements, speak to your doctor.

Fats and Fatty Acids

Fats are long-chained molecules constructed from the fatty acids and glycerol. Both are obtained from our diets. Fats are found in both animals and plants. They can be saturated (those found in red meats) or unsaturated (plants and fish). Saturated fats have high melting points and are therefore solid at room temperature (eg lard and butter). In contrast, unsaturated fats have low melting points and form oils at room temperature (eg 'vegetable oil', peanut oil and olive oil).

Today, saturated fats are accepted as being 'unhealthy', predisposing us, as they do, to heart attacks, strokes, diabetes, gall-stones and certain types of cancer. However, you have to be very careful about the 'polyunsaturated products' that you buy. Butter is hard because it contains a lot of saturated fats. Butter substitutes contain polyunsaturated fats but saturated fats must also be present for the margarine to be speadable – pouring margarine on your toast would not be a very successful marketing concept! Unfortunately, some margarines have such a high saturated fat content that they are not significantly different from butter. When buying polyunsaturated products, choose those articles which claim to be extra low in fat (eg low fat cream and butters and skimmed milk), but check the contents list for the proportion of saturates and polyunsaturates.

Grilling and microwaving food provide healthy alternatives to frying either with a saturated fat (lard or butter) or a polyunsaturate (vegetable oil). It is easy to make body fat but much harder to lose it again! Most of the excess energy from carbohydrates that is not immediately used or stored as glycogen is converted into fat. Fats, however, cannot be converted into carbohydrates. Fats are a great energy source and are evolution's answer to storing energy on a long-term basis.

Unfortunately, because the process of turning fat into energy is relatively slow and can only take place when sugar is being 'burnt', as far as our training programme is concerned, fat is really only of use to us in the endurance marches, endurance cycling and the marathon and ultra marathon. This is one of the reasons why once you have laid down fat it is so difficult to get rid of it! In the West, up to 30 per cent of our energy comes in the form of fats and much of this becomes stored in deposits under the skin. In contrast, the leaner peoples of the Third World have diets which are composed of 10 per cent fat or less. The SAS and all serious athletes aim for this lower figure. This does require a special effort on your part and a very carefully chosen diet, where skimmed milk is substituted for whole-fat milk; margarine is eaten instead of butter; cottage cheese is exchanged for Cheddar; sausages and hamburgers, if eaten at all, are grilled; lard is rejected in favour of vegetable oil, and fish and chicken replace meat. Remember, even unsaturated fats should be eaten in minimal quantities. In the same way as there are essential amino acids, there are essential polyunsaturated fatty acids (PUFAs). These are only present in fish and plant oils. The best sources are sunflower and safflower seed oils, cod liver oil and the meat of herrings, mackerel and salmon. The PUFAs have two main jobs. Firstly, they are essential to the well-being of all tissue and organs. Secondly, they play a vital role in the synthesis of body chemicals called prostaglandins, which in turn play important roles in tissue-healing and repair.

As with amino acids, it is possible to buy fatty-acid supplements for athletes. The biochemical process that leads to the synthesis of the prostaglandins is long and slow – extremely so in some people. In recognition of this, doctors have recommended that some athletes take supplements of gamma-linolenic acid during their peak training periods. Current medical advice concerning fats can be summarised as follows:

♦ Not more than 30 per cent of your daily energy should come from fats.
♦ Athletes, elite soldiers and anybody seriously interested in keeping fit and remaining healthy should aim at the lower figure of 10 per cent. This target can only be attained with willpower and a careful diet.
♦ Unsaturated fats should be substituted for saturated fats at every opportunity, but be careful of the pitfalls.
♦ The essential polyunsaturated fatty acids cannot be synthesised by the body. They are available from fish oils, some fish meat and plant oils.
♦ Gamma-linolenic acid may be beneficial during peak training periods.

Cholesterol and Heart Disease

The subject of cholesterol intake and its role in heart disease is complex and controversial. Part of the problem is that we produce our own cholesterol and the body tends to make more as the amount in our diet is reduced. However, all the experts accept that too much cholesterol leads to heart disease since it tends to clog the arteries, particularly the artery which supplies blood to the heart itself.

Cholesterol is present in meat and dairy products but particularly high levels are present in eggs. Indeed, some surgeons have been known to grade the severity of their patient's disease in terms of their likely egg consumption! Removing the fat from meat, grilling meat, avoiding hamburgers and sausages, reducing your intake of dairy products and eating no more than one or two eggs each week should reduce your cholesterol consumption. There are other factors promoting heart disease. Current medical recommendations include: stop smoking; it damages both the heart and the insides of the arteries.

- If your blood pressure is high, take steps to reduce it. Work with your doctor to identify those factors in your diet or lifestyle that may be contributing to your high blood pressure. If all else fails, ensure that you are prescribed the appropriate hypotensive drugs.
- Aim for a balanced lifestyle with the minimum of stress. Remember, your life is in the hands of the people who make you angry.
- Take regular, moderate exercise, with sessions lasting 30 minutes or more. This conditions your heart. Exercise on its own is not the answer. If you do not correct predisposing factors in your diet and lifestyle, even regular marathons will not protect you against coronary heart disease and atherosclerosis.

Complex and Simple Sugars

The complex sugars present in animal muscle (glycogen) and root crops and cereals (starch) are long, branched chains, built by adding many simple sugars together. The complex sugars are just a good way of storing sugar until it is needed. In humans and animals, glycogen is broken down in the muscles to produce the simple sugar, glucose, which serves as the 'fuel for life'.

Glucose levels in the blood are carefully regulated to ensure that the muscles, brain and other organs are constantly bathed in this energy-producing sugar. Simple sugars, such as glucose, taste sweet and dissolve in water. They are found naturally in fruits, fruit juices and honey. Simple and complex sugars are all part of a group of similar chemicals called carbohydrates. The simple sugars can be single molecules such as glucose, which are known as monosaccharides, or double molecules such as fructose, the predominant sugar in bananas known as disaccharides, while the complex sugars are called polysaccharides. Rather than high-fat and high-protein diets which are unhealthy and frowned upon, the person in training needs a high-carbohydrate diet. Some 50 to 60 per cent of our energy intake should come from sugars. However, these should be the complex carbohydrates, such as starch – and to a certain extent glycogen from animal muscle – and not the simple sugars.

The simple sugars rot teeth, and large amounts taken over a short period can damage the liver. They can produce a very high blood sugar level, and as this is brought under control, the blood sugar level can then 'rebound' to very low levels, resulting in shaking, dizziness and general weakness.

The other problem with simple sugars is that sugar-rich convenience foods such as chocolate, crisps, ice-cream, biscuits, cake, and popcorn, to name just a few, are not only rich in sugar but they are also rich in fat. The convenience foods are therefore self-defeating since the whole point of a high-carbohydrate diet is to obtain our energy from sugars instead of fats!

Competitive sportsmen and women 'load' their muscle glycogen before an important sports event. The muscles of sedentary people are limited as to the amount of glycogen that can be stored. After hard exercise, however, very much more sugar can be stored in the muscles as glycogen. What happens is that two to three hours after hard, intensive exercise, the sugar stores are depleted and the athlete's body begins to burn fatty acids. So, for a brief time after exercise, fat metabolism takes care of all the athlete's energy needs. If, at this point, the athlete eats a high-carbohydrate meal, almost all of the available sugar goes into the muscles as glycogen.

The meal recommended by doctors for professional athletes is cereal with a little skimmed milk and the syrup from canned fruit, washed down with a high-energy glucose drink. Very little fat is present in this meal and the fruit syrup replaces the potassium lost in sweat. Also note that the emphasis here is on starch rather than the simple sugars. Complex sugars have to be broken down in our bowels. They are therefore absorbed more slowly and are less likely to cause wild fluctuations in blood sugar levels.

There are some complex carbohydrates, for example cellulose, that we cannot digest. Animals such as sheep and cows only manage to use cellulose as an energy source because they have bacteria in their guts which digest this complex sugar for them. These indigestible carbohydrates are important in our diets too. We call them 'fibre'. Fibre adds bulk to our food and gives that satisfying feeling of being full without over-eating! Fibre also keeps the bowels moving and prevents the harmful build-up of the chemicals which could cause cancer. Finally, fibre absorbs water and so softens our stools, thus preventing the bowel damage and haemorrhoids which result from straining to expel our stools.

Fruits and plant products are high in fibre, but a word of caution. Because these indigestible carbohydrates cannot supply us with energy, and in absorbing water tend to extend the bowel, high-fibre foods should not form a significant part of our diets during periods of peak training. In other words, the amount of fibre in our diets should vary with the intensity of our training and consequent energy requirements.

In Summary

- Some 50–60 per cent of our energy should come from sugars.
- The complex carbohydrates such as starch are better sources of energy than the simple sugars.
- After intensive exercise, the muscles can be loaded with glycogen by eating a meal rich in sugar.
- Carbohydrate-rich diets are beneficial during intensive training.
- Indigestible sugars or 'fibre' should form an important part of our diet but not during periods of peak training.

Vitamins

Vitamins are a range of chemicals needed by the body but usually in quite small amounts. They have various roles but most perform some vital function in body chemistry. It is generally accepted that people on well-balanced diets do not require vitamin supplements. On the other hand, athletes on high-carbohydrate or other unusual diets may require regular vitamin supplements. Vitamins come in two varieties, depending on whether they dissolve in water or fat. The fat-soluble vitamins (A, D, E and K) are stored in our body fat and are slowly released as the fat is broken down to be used as energy. In contrast, the water-soluble vitamins (C and B) cannot be stored in the body and are required in regular daily amounts.

Vitamin A: Vitamin A is found in animal fats and fish oils such as cod liver oil. Deficiency is associated with increased infections, night blindness and stunted growth. It is important in the maintenance of healthy skin. It is also a powerful anti-oxidant and part of the body's defence against free radicals. Free radicals have assumed more importance recently as the food industry has started to irradiate food to extend its shelf-life. Radiation produces free radicals.

The World Health Organisation, concerned by this problem, has estimated that around one third of the world's population is deficient in this vitamin. Nevertheless, in the West, athletes and sportsmen/women on well-balanced diets are very unlikely to be deficient in vitamin A. Cod liver oil is a very good source not only of vitamin A but the essential polyunsaturated fatty acids. However, a word of caution! Over-dosing on vitamin A will result in fatal liver damage. Polar bear liver is an extremely rich source of this vitamin and has been responsible for the deaths of certain polar explorers.

Trappers in seventeenth century Canada were often forced to survive the winter on the flesh and offal of trapped animals. Although food was in plentiful supply, many died under mysterious circumstances and it is now believed that hypervitaminosis A was responsible.

Vitamin D: This vitamin is found in fish oil and dairy products but is also synthesised in the skin in bright sunlight. Vitamin D deficiency, which can result in a condition known as 'rickets', is only seen in heavily-clothed people living in areas enjoying very little sunshine.

Vitamin E: A deficiency of this vitamin may affect a person's ability to reach peak performance. It is important in the maintenance and repair of muscle and improves the amount of anaerobic energy that can be generated in muscles. There is no evidence, however, that increased intake of vitamin E improves overall performance. Animal fats and dairy products, particularly eggs, are good sources of this vitamin.

Vitamin C: Vitamin C has been postulated to help the body fight infections and even protect against cancer. However, expert opinion remains divided. It is certainly involved in the maintenance and healing of soft tissue. Vitamin C is water-soluble and a dose of around 60 mg is required each day from our diet. Fruit and green vegetables are rich sources of this vitamin.

Vitamin B: This is really a complex of some 12 water-soluble vitamins. The better known include thiamine, riboflavin, niacin, pantothenic acid, pyridoxine, the cobalamins, the folates, biotin and inositol. Many of these substances are involved in sugar metabolism and even mild deficiencies may be expected adversely to affect training. Sources of the major B vitamins include:

Thiamine (B1)	Wheat germ, oatmeal and yeast.
Riboflavin (B2)	Yeasts, peas and beans.
Niacin	Many plant and animal foods.
Pyridoxine (B6)	Synthesised in the liver from common, naturally-occurring precursors.
Folate	Green vegetables and meat.
Cobalamins (B12)	Meat and animal products.
Biotin	Eggs and dairy products.
Pantothenic acid	Many animal and plant sources.
Vitamin K	Synthesised by bacteria in our intestines. Also present in green leafy vegetables, meat and dairy products. Plays an important role in blood clotting.

The current medical advice to sportsmen and women on vitamin intake can be summarised as follows:

- Vitamin deficiency can adversely affect training, but most well-balanced diets contain sufficient vitamins.
- There may be an increased demand for some vitamins during peak training periods.
- Oral contraceptives and smoking increase the body's demand for vitamins B, C and E.
- Vitamin supplements are also beneficial for those on carbohydrate-rich diets. The fat-soluble vitamins should be taken before peak training, while the water-soluble ones should be taken daily during peak training.
- A greatly increased intake of vitamins will not improve performance and, in the case of vitamin A, could have fatal consequences.

Minerals

Some 15 trace elements perform a range of important functions in the body and are required in varying amounts. During peak training sessions, some minerals may be lost and will need to be replaced either by supplements or from the diet.

Sodium and Potassium: There is ample sodium in the human body but potassium is lost in sweat during intense training. It can be replaced by eating fruit or drinking fruit juice.

Calcium: Calcium phosphate is responsible for the rigidity of bone. It is not 'lost' within the bone but is continually turning over. A higher flux occurs during strenuous activity. Calcium also has a vital role in muscle contraction. Inevitably, some calcium is lost from the body and needs to be replaced. The major source is dairy products such as milk and cheese. Removing the fat, eg by skimming milk, does not reduce the calcium content.

Copper: Copper is important in a wide range of functions, including protecting the body from the sorts of minor injury which occur during peak training. Very little copper is flushed from the body with the urine, but it is lost in sweat. Moderate supplements should be considered after endurance exercises or after training in a hot gym or outdoors in full sunshine.

Chromium: This mineral is an important co-factor in sugar chemistry. Studies have shown that athletes lose twice as much chromium in their urine after exercise than on rest days.

Iron: Iron deficiency results in anaemia, and even mild anaemias reduce the potential to undertake aerobic exercise. Anaemia can result from loss of blood, too little iron in the diet, impaired iron absorption from the intestine or some other problem in blood synthesis. There is usually more than sufficient iron in the well-balanced diet, but it can become limited in diets lacking red meat and green vegetables. Women who experience prolonged menstrual bleeding may never have sufficient iron in their diets, particularly if they are vegetarian or vegan.

Liver is a particularly good source of iron and a good natural dietary supplement. Iron supplements should be taken under medical advice since they can be dangerous. Anyone suspecting that they are either anaemic or iron- deficient should consult their doctor.

Magnesium: Magnesium is intimately associated with energy production in the body. It is widely present in food, particularly green plants. Ample amounts should be present in almost all diets. Nevertheless, studies have shown that blood magnesium levels drop after heavy exercise.

Selenium: Selenium is required in extremely small amounts but is essential. It is a vital co-factor for the anti-oxidant enzyme, glutathione peroxidase. This enzyme helps repair tissue damage, which can occur during vigorous exercise, and it also helps to protect the body by mopping up free radicals.

Zinc: Zinc is an important co-factor for more than 100 enzymes, including those involved in energy production in the muscles. Approximately 60 per cent of zinc in the human body is found in the muscles. Some athletes take zinc supplements. It is recommended that intake should be started just before, and continued throughout, peak training.

- Most mineral requirements are present in well-balanced diets.
- Those undertaking hard, strenuous exercise may benefit from mineral supplements. Proprietary brands are easily available in the high street but should probably only be taken during periods of peak training.
- High-dose or regular iron supplements should only be taken after consultation with your doctor.

Fluids

Fluids are a vital accompaniment to training. A marathon runner, allowed to eat and drink at will, can expect to lose up to eight per cent of his or her body weight and 13–14 per cent of his or her total body water in the course of the race. Most of the water is lost through sweat and this serves to concentrate the salts in his or her tissues. It was thought at one time that warm fluids prevented cramping and that a large volume of fluid was emptied from the stomach more quickly than a smaller volume to find its way into the blood. In fact, doctors have discovered that small quantities (100–200 ml or ¼–⅓ pt) of a cold drink, taken four to five times an hour, both restore body water and cool the body more effectively than either ingesting larger amounts of fluids or warm fluids.

In summary, small, regular amounts of cold water or a weak glucose solution dramatically restores body water and minimises the risk of dehydration. During exercise, keep away from sugar-rich fizzy drinks. You can start drinking rich, syrupy, energy-packed drinks two to three hours after training, when your water balance has returned to normal. Most importantly, on peak exercise days, keep away from alcohol, which switches off the hormone responsible for controlling water loss. Alcohol also seriously disturbs the mechanism which controls blood sugar; the two major components of a hangover are dehydration and too little sugar in the blood.

Seven-Day Menu

If we eat a hearty breakfast, we should only need a light lunch and this will give us a good appetite for our evening meal. When training, the last meal of the day should be eaten in the early evening. A large supper which leaves you feeling bloated is not exactly conducive to a good sleep.

Breakfast: Cereal with milk (skimmed or semi-skimmed if you are watching those fats!), scrambled egg cooked in the microwave, toast made from wholemeal bread, grilled lean, unsmoked bacon, baked beans, tomatoes (tinned or grilled), mushrooms (microwaved).

Lunch: A salad with fresh vegetables. Fruit to follow (optional).

Dinner: It is possible to eat a varied diet every evening which is also nourishing, healthy and tasty. I recommend that red meat is only eaten once or twice a week. Poultry and fish are very enjoyable substitutes. Rabbit is another meat which contains little fat and is tasty and cheap.

Monday	Roast chicken (with skin removed)
Tuesday	Steamed fish
Wednesday	Pasta with lean mince (red meat!)
Thursday	Liver, lightly grilled
Friday	Stewed rabbit
Saturday	Grilled steak with fat removed
Sunday	Roast turkey

Eat these meals with as many vegetables as you like, but try not to use butter and oil when cooking them. You can introduce a wide variety of vegetables into your diet by eating salads. A little vinegar and water will add to the taste. Try to avoid mayonnaise and oil-based dressings.

Health Foods

Garlic: This fascinating vegetable is purported to have great medicinal properties. It is said to lower blood pressure and it contains significant amounts of the water-soluble vitamins, B and C, as well as calcium, phosphorus and potassium. It lends an excellent flavour to meals but unfortunately it taints the breath. If taken in sufficiently large quantities, the volatile chemicals responsible for the smell are excreted in sweat, thus producing a fascinating body aroma! Garlic tablets are an excellent alternative to fresh garlic and are odourless.

Kelp: Kelp is dried and powdered seaweed. It contains a wide range of minerals, including sodium chloride, so take it sparingly. It is also a natural source of iodine – vital for thyroid function – and is often recommended for people living in areas where natural sources of iodine are lacking.

The Yeasts: Yeast is an excellent source of protein and the B complex of vitamins. It is also rich in iron. Yeast supplements are said to lower cholesterol and generally perk up your system!

Alfalfa: The green leaves of this legume contain a range of essential amino acids and vitamins. Alfalfa is a good source of vitamin K, which is a necessary co-factor in blood clotting. The leaves of the plant are said to be beneficial in stomach disorders and to perk up a jaded appetite. It is available in tablet form.

Ginseng: For thousands of years, the Chinese have used ginseng to stimulate mental and physical energy. Critics, however, argue that gingseng's 'feel-good factor' is due to its high alcohol content and the presence of the stimulant drug, ephedrine. So take it sparingly! Nevertheless, it has been reported to be beneficial for people with blood and circulation problems. It is available in both capsule and liquid preparations.

Yucca: The Native Americans of the southern United States and Central America have used the ground, succulent leaves of the Yucca 'tuft-tree' as a general herbal remedy for a wide range of ailments. Today, it is generally accepted to possess many health-giving properties and there is some evidence that it has anti-inflammatory properties useful in the treatment of arthritis. For those of us living outside the deserts of the Americas, it is available in tablet form from health-food stores and suppliers.

Yoghurt: Yoghurt is a dairy product which contains a living culture of harmless bacteria. It is believed to possess general health-giving properties. Some people, particularly Africans, lack the gut enzyme, lactase, which breaks down the milk sugar, lactose. In the absence of this enzyme, the sugar in milk passes into the large intestine where it is fermented by intestinal bacteria, producing severe flatulence and diarrhoea. This 'allergy to milk' can be overcome if it is drunk after a meal of yoghurt, since the bacteria in the yoghurt supply the missing enzyme!

CHAPTER TWELVE

Your Own SAS Diet

Service in the SAS is very different from that in other units of the British Army. Frequently posted abroad to very remote areas, the Regiment has learnt to eat and enjoy the local food. During operations alongside local tribes, SAS patrols had to become more adventurous and be prepared to savour local delicacies such as grubs, snakes and the occasional monkey. This was often a welcome change to the good old army 'compo', and an alternative to the freeze-dried, light-weight rations issued to Special Forces. As you can imagine, the light-weight rations were unbelievably monotonous, forcing the lads to become good cooks and to learn how to disguise the bland taste with spices and flavourings. In time, SAS-style curries and stews became favourites with the Regiment.

Back in Hereford, SAS food is second to none. There is always a wide choice of meals and the mess hall has a 'help yourself' policy. Not many of the lads have a weight problem and it is a work-out in itself carrying the heavily laden plates back to your table!

Eating SAS-Style

On operations we would only eat one meal a day. Breakfast and lunch were just a brew and a hardtack biscuit – if you were lucky! You were always hungry on operations and you just had to make up for it when you got back to base. These eating habits are still part of my life. Get out of bed early and go for a run. This is best done on an empty stomach.

An early morning run not only invigorates the system, it also gets the body used to working from its own reserves of energy. When you are working as hard as we were, you need an energy intake of around 5,000 calories per day. That is a lot of food! Consequently, it becomes even more important to eat sensibly, avoiding cholesterol-rich foods and limiting delicacies such as cakes, sweets and ice cream. We soon learnt at Hereford that it was better to eat little and often rather than trying to pack all of your energy requirements into one meal.

Get into the habit of fasting one day in seven. It gives your system a well-earned rest. On your fast day, drink plenty of water. You can still exercise, but avoid taxing routines such as endurance work. In fasting, we are also learning how to go without one of the things we take for granted. It helps you develop both your body and your willpower. It takes discipline to fast each week and self-discipline is a large part of the overall ethos of the SAS.

The day after your fast, give yourself a treat and choose the meal that you most fancy. Little pleasures give you something to look forward to and help break the rigours and frustrations of training.

Let us now have a look at some SAS meals. These would certainly not be included in a weight-watcher's diet. On the contrary, they are meals for fit, well-conditioned people, engaged in heavy work or training to the limits of their endurance.

Ranger Porridge
Ranger porridge was a favourite in the jungle.
● Boil the oats in a little water until they are cooked and then
● Pour a little condensed milk over the top.

After this porridge, you would be able to slay dragons! Follow this with eggs and bacon – not a full-blown London Grill!

Fat Boy's Breakfast
The 'Fat Boy' starts with bacon and egg.
● Be sure that you cut the fat off the bacon, which should be grilled not fried.
● Scramble the eggs, or you could boil them.
● Add tomatoes, baked beans, mushrooms and kidneys.
● Prepare one or two slices of wholemeal toast to soak up the juices.
● A glass of fruit juice will wash it all down nicely.

NAAFI Break
At 10 am, we always had a NAAFI break at Hereford. This was so welcome that, for me, it has become a hard habit to break. Tea and toast were the order of the day. In fact, I think the best drink of the day is a

nice mug of tea with a large spoon of condensed milk. But remember, tea contains a diuretic, so limit yourself to one cup at each meal. With an eye to those 5,000 calories, you could substitute a filled roll for the toast. Fillings such as tuna, egg, salmon, or ham should ensure plenty of variety. Lunch was at 1 pm and was usually a soup, salad or sandwiches.

'A' Squadron Salad
- Cut up the lettuce into fine strips and add diced carrots, onions, peppers, tomatoes, cheese, nuts or any other vegetable you might fancy.
- Add tuna or ham, and eat as much as you want!

'B' Squadron Soup
- Dice potatoes and add them to a small volume of water.
- Add diced swede, broccoli, onions, carrots, leeks, courgettes, mushrooms, beans, peas and lentils (as required).
- Simmer until the vegetables are tender.

Boat Troop Chowder
Use any fish that you fancy.

- Fillet carefully, removing all the bones.
- Bring to the boil in a large saucepan, adding winkles, cockles, mussels, whelks, shrimps, prawns or any other seafood you like.
- Finally, add hot chilli sauce to taste.

Pea and Ham Soup: Lofty's favourite!
This is a real rib-clinger!
- Boil a bacon joint until it is well cooked.
- Allow to cool.
- Skim the fat off the water and add potatoes and lentils.

When eating salads, prepare only enough for one meal. Do not store it. Buy as you need it and eat it fresh. Cook all soups in portions large enough for a couple of meals. You can store these in the fridge but they are not suitable for home freezing. Make sure they are re-heated thoroughly. I prefer to use a microwave. Have a snack around 3 pm. I like a mug of tea and a sandwich.

Curries

There are very few dishes more appetising than curry. You could eat a different curry every day of the week and each would have its own distinctive flavour. The great thing with curry is that you never get fed up with it. You can curry almost anything: fish, meats or just vegetables. The SAS are masters at creating new curries!

SAS CURRY

Use whatever meat is at hand, in true SAS style, to create this nutritious and warming dish.

- Finely chop one or more cloves of garlic according to taste.
- Add finely chopped onions and stir-fry both with a small amount of oil in a wok or frying pan. When available, I prefer to use olive oil, or banana or coconut oil.
- Add curry powder, or better, curry paste. Use according to taste but never more than a tablespoon.
- Fry in oil. It is important to fry the curry powder otherwise it will not blend into the meal and it will taste gritty. If you like hot curries, you can add one or more chillies.
- When the curry powder has been well mixed with the oil, add the meat and stir-fry until golden brown.
- Add tomato puree to taste.
- Finally, add your stock and simmer for a few hours.
- Serve the curry on a bed of rice.

ULU CHICKEN CURRY

If you have never tasted this type of curry, you are in for a treat!

- Place a whole chicken, including the neck and giblets, in a large saucepan of water and bring to the boil.
- Cook for 20 minutes and then remove the saucepan from the stove.
- Fillet the chicken, removing all the skin and bones.
- Stir-fry onions, garlic and curry powder and then add the chicken meat and cook until it is lightly browned.
- Finally, add pineapple and cream of coconut.

SELECTION FISH CURRY
Any large fish will suffice for this dish.

- Boil the whole fish in plenty of lightly salted water with a drop of lemon juice and a little hot chilli sauce.
- Stir-fry onions and garlic before adding curry powder and spoonful of garam masala.
- Peel the flesh off the fish and add it to the wok.
- Retain the water as stock.
- Stir-fry until the flesh is a light brown.
- Add prawns and cook for several minutes.
- Finally, mix with the stock and serve with rice.

Rice
Cooking rice is an art form. Here are a few useful tips:

- Wash the rice thoroughly in three changes of water.
- Fill a large saucepan with water and add a pinch of salt.
- Bring the water to the boil.
- Add the rice to the boiling water and allow to boil for several minutes.
- Turn the heat down and allow to simmer until the rice softens.
- Hold the saucepan under the cold water tap and empty the rice into a colander, washing it as you do so. This separates the grains and makes the rice fluffy.

NASI GORENG
This is the Malay name for fried rice. It is a great favourite among older members of the Regiment.

- Boil the rice, making sure to wash and strain well.
- Pour a little oil into a wok or large saucepan.
- Stir-fry garlic and onions, tomatoes, peppers and one or two chillies.
- Add thin strips of beef and ham, and prawns.
- Add rice and mix well.
- Add three whisked eggs.
- Stir the food, mixing well, until it is cooked.
- Finally, add two tablespoons of soy sauce.

A Steak Recipe

There is nothing quite like a juicy steak after a hard training session. Use this recipe to give yourself a treat.

- Choose a thick cut of lean steak. Fillet or rump steak will do nicely.
- Trim off any fat and rub lightly with garlic.
- Cook under a hot grill or barbecue over a bed of hot charcoal.
- Turn for one minute or until the meat is nicely brown. This seals in all the juices.
- Turn down the heat and cook it slowly to order.

Puddings

Try to develop a taste for savoury rather than sweet foods. On your rest day, eat what you like, but during the rest of the week avoid cakes, chocolates and sweets. The best pudding is yoghurt, followed by fresh fruit.

Water

Drink plenty of water. If you fit a filter to your tap, you can save a fortune on bottled water. A very refreshing drink can be made by squeezing lime or lemon into water and then adding a spoonful of honey.

Isotonic Drinks

Isotonic drinks containing salts are a good way of replacing the blood electrolytes which are lost in sweat. Isotonic drinks contain not only vital salts, such as potassium, but sugar to replace the lost energy. Take these before and after heavy exercise and they will help your body recover quickly. There are no magic potions that will build fitness and toughness. What we are looking for does not come in a bottle. It is tough, it is hard but only the best wear the sand-coloured beret of the SAS.

REMEMBER: Who cares wins!

CHAPTER THIRTEEN

Survival Food

Rations are always a problem. As rucksacks get heavier, a vicious circle develops; any increase in weight means that a person has to do more work and therefore needs more energy-producing food. The SAS Regiment has solved this problem by expecting its members to survive on light rations or, where necessary, live off the land.

The other problem is that on operations, vital equipment has to be crammed into every pocket and every corner of the bergens. There is often little or no space for rations. There is only so much you can carry! Even under ideal conditions, a soldier can only carry water and rations for about four days, and we could be out in the field for weeks at a time.

SAS-Style Rations

The little food that can be carried must be of a high calorific value for its size and weight. Tins and bottles are out!

The SAS soldier carries freeze-dried and dehydrated rations. Freeze-dried foods are the better, being more palatable. Dehydrated food lacks both texture and taste, and the process of removing the water from the food also removes vitamins and minerals, although these are sometimes put back later. Freeze-dried food can be either eaten as a 'munch' or reconstituted.

A wide range of menus are available, offering meats such as beef, lamb, chicken and pork. Complete meals are also available from outlets specialising in supplying equipment for mountaineering and outdoor activities.

Among the meals offered are real delicacies such as spaghetti bolognaise, chicken supreme and lamb tikka. These can be very tasty if you follow the simple cooking instructions. Usually, you are told to add a measure of boiling water to the bag and then stir until the food is fully reconstituted. Even puddings such as creamed rice and apples and custard are available. Not bad when you are living rough on the hills!

One important piece of kit must find a place in your pack and that is your brew kit. There is nothing like a hot drink to kick-start your whole system into action after a long, cold night on the hills or a punishing hike in driving rain or snow.

More importantly, warm drinks keep hypothermia at bay and are great for the morale! A nice cup of tea will pour stimulating caffeine into your veins, while stock cubes and hot chocolate are almost meals in themselves. On hot days, isotonic drinks and lemonade powders offer a pleasant alternative to luke-warm water.

On operations, SAS patrols eat one meal a day. Often, lunch is an energy-rich snack that can be eaten quickly during a five-minute rest stop. Nuts and raisins, dates, dried fruit, Mars bars, oat bars and Kendall Mint Cake are all packed with energy. A high blood glucose level will be really appreciated when the going gets tough.

In really cold weather, when you are using a lot of energy just to keep warm, or when time is not pressing, you can always enjoy a hot cup of soup. Powdered soups come in all varieties, they taste good and are packed with energy and nutrients. Breakfast should be simple and hot. A warm, sweet cup of something and a biscuit may be all the breakfast you need. A 'full breakfast' could be oats and reconstituted milk, powdered egg or biscuits and cheese. But remember, what you pack into your rucksack will have to be carried, so get used to living simply!

The main meal of the day became a real ritual for us. We spent a long time preparing it since we knew it would be our last good meal for another 24 hours. Everybody found a place for their packets of spice. They really made the curry and rice come alive!

The way to prepare your rations for short and long-term expeditions is to use the 'brick system'. Divide your total rations into three different types of 'bricks', each containing around 1,500 calories. Brick 'A' is the lightweight ration. It can be eaten with the very minimum of preparation and no cooking should be required.

Brick 'A' Rations
Cheese and biscuits
Chocolate or *Mars* bars
Nut and oat bars
Nuts and raisins

Boiled sweets
Oats and dried fruit
Isotonic drinks or powdered lemonade
Meat 'bars' such as Pepperoni, cured sausage or beef jerky
Sweet biscuits

These are just some of the foods you might think of putting in your light-weight rations. This type of 'brick' will form the majority of your rations when you are climbing, canoeing or on the move across the hills.

Brick 'B'

This type of ration complements the lightweight rations and it either forms the main meal of the day or the meals you would eat in a forward base camp. These rations require cooking and therefore time-consuming preparation. Once again, each 'brick' should offer a 1,500-calorie meal. The sort of food you would expect to find in these rations would include:

Complete one-course main meals
Puddings
Egg powder, oats and biscuits (breakfast)
Energy-rich bars, nuts and raisins and/or soups (lunch)
Tea, milk and sugar and/or stock cubes

As with the lightweight rations, this is only a guide. Be creative and pack the goodies you most like to eat.

Brick 'C'

These are the little luxuries that you may choose to carry. Although these are 'luxuries', each 'brick' should still contain around 1,500 calories, giving you value for weight. On a long expedition, these rations can make a welcome change to your diet. Typical foods to be considered are:

Chocolate drinks
Egg powder
Potato powder
Rice and/or pasta
Dried onions, garlic and spices
Flapjacks
Biscuits
High-energy bars
Sweet and savoury spreads

These rations are designed to make life a little more pleasant, even under the very worst of conditions.

Choosing and Packing Your 'Bricks'

With your rations divided into the three types, you can now decide how you will mix and match them to suit the particular activity you are planning.

On a short, three-day outing, when you know you will be constantly on the move, I suggest that you carry three 'A' bricks and one 'B' brick. On a seven-day hike across the hills, you will need something more substantial and you could opt for seven As, three Bs and one C.

The beauty of this system is that the choice is yours and the combinations are endless! You should find almost everything you need to put these rations together on the shelves of your local supermarket. Of course, you should adapt each ration to your planned activity, the area to which you are going and the time of year.

In winter, or in cold, wet areas such as the mountains, the main problem will be keeping warm. Your rations should reflect this need and should contain more fatty foods, starch-rich foods such as rice and potatoes and 'instant-energy', sugar-rich foods such as Mars bars. Make sure that you also pack enough ingredients for plenty of warm drinks.

In summer or in hot, dry terrains you will not want to carry an over-loaded Bergen in the energy-sapping heat. Keeping warm will not be a problem, so you will need fewer calories. You can afford to carry a high proportion of lightweight rations. This will be a mercy if you cannot find water sources along your route, since you may have to carry water with you! Remember that you will lose a lot of body salt in sweat, so carry some isotonic drinks, a little table salt to put on your food and some fruit juice to replace that all-important lost potassium.

When you have put your food together into 'bricks', make sure that you pack them well. Place all individual items in strong polythene bags, then fold over the tops and heat-seal them with a warm iron. Finally, seal all the individual items in a large polythene bag and mark it clearly 'A', 'B' or 'C'. You will also need various sundry items such as matches, salt, chewing gum and toilet paper. These, too, should be sealed in polythene bags and then placed in an outer pocket or on the top of your rucksack.

Stoves

In the military, we used to cook our grub on solid hexamine blocks. These were not very good. I mention them because they are exactly the sort of solid-fuel cooker to avoid! Hexamine burns with a relatively 'cold', smoky, yellow flame. In a wind, most of the heat was blown away, although that was sometimes a blessing as the fumes were toxic! The fumes also had a very distinctive smell that could spread quite a long way, persisting on the still, moist air under the tree canopy.

Later, some members of the Regiment carried liquid gas stoves. Unlike hexamine, these burnt with a hot, smokeless flame but they were far from perfect. There were two problems. Firstly, you had much the same problem with the wind taking away the heat from the bottom of your mess tin. Secondly, at high altitudes the gas is released at a reduced pressure and, consequently, does not burn as well. I prefer the Coleman's solid-fuel stoves which avoid these problems.

The Peak One Multi-Fuel Stove can burn Coleman's Fuel or paraffin and one filling will burn for up to six hours. The windshield and pan support on this cooker are designed to direct 80 per cent of the available heat towards the mess tin. The manufacturers advertise their Peak One Multi-Fuel Stove as an expedition cooker, able to operate efficiently under quite adverse conditions. Coleman also market a slightly cheaper stove which can burn either Coleman's Fuel or petrol. The Peak One Petrol Stove also comes with a sturdy tripod and a windshield which directs most of the available heat at your mess tin.

Once again, the fuel tank is quite large and the stove comes equipped with a pump, fuel lever and self-cleaner. The Petrol Stove is advertised as ideal for 'brewing up on the summit of Pen-Y-Fan on a sunny day'. However, as I always seem to miss the sunny days on Pen-Y-Fan, I tend to lean towards the slightly more expensive Peak One Multi-Fuel Stove. Mini cookers have some of the disadvantages of the old hexamine cooker but they make good survival cookers and can be slipped into a pouch on your belt kit. Like the hexamine cookers, they are small, cheap and burn solid fuel at a relatively low temperature. There the similarities end. Most mini-cookers burn alcohol jelly which produces a smokeless, non-toxic, odourless flame. This means that they can be used inside a survival shelter or tent. This is a great boon in bad weather.

A new cooker comes equipped with enough fuel to burn continuously for about two hours. Refills burn for around 90 minutes.

3 MENTAL AGILITY

CHAPTER FOURTEEN
Positive Thinking

Positive thinking is the key to success in dealing with dangerous or frightening situations. We have to be positive in our approach to life; we have to believe in ourselves. In order to achieve these aims, we have to work to eliminate weaknesses within ourselves and practice those skills at which we do not excel. Life in a competitive world is hard and it has a way of exploiting flaws in our characters. Be aware of your limitations and resolve to do something about them.

Motivation

To even embark on a fitness programme requires motivation. Poor health may supply the necessary motivation. You can easily become fed up with shortness of breath or constantly feeling tired. We can all improve ourselves, our lifestyles and our jobs and it starts with recognising our weaknesses and problems in our lives.

Compare yourself with other people of the same age and sex. Are they healthier and happier than you? Select a person who you admire greatly and ask yourself what it is that you admire about them. You will have many of the same qualities although, perhaps, somewhat less developed. If this was not true, you would not admire these qualities; other people are mirrors in which we can see ourselves.

However, do not merely copy other people, analyse what it is that you like about them and concentrate on developing these qualities in your own life. Equally, analyse the weaknesses of others and ask yourself if you have these weaknesses too.

Study the mistakes that happen in life and ask why they happened. Common problems occur commonly. If you learn what has gone wrong now, you may be able to put it right in the future. It is human to make mistakes but incredibly foolish to go through life repeating the same mistakes! The world only ever seems to remember the winners. Nobody likes to be in second place, but to be a winner you first have to be a loser.

People who have been training hard for most of their lives will be fitter, stronger and faster than you. Learn from them. Study their training routines, seek their advice on diets and talk to them about how they motivate themselves.

Once you have begun your training programme, you can start to experiment with different diets and exercise routines to suit you. We are all different and we all have individual needs. Think hard about your goals and then go for them! Use your training programme and your job to help structure your life. Set yourself sensible goals and celebrate when you achieve them. Seek an independent assessment of your training programme. It is all too easy to get stuck in the rut of doing only those activities at which you excel. Ask your best friend or a training companion to comment on your standard. Ask their advice on how they would modify your training programme. Share your life experiences and problems with them.

Criticism can be painful but, providing that it is constructive criticism, it can enable you to see yourself as other people see you. There will be times when you will be tested by life. Things will go wrong and you must be prepared for this to happen. Always have contingency plans. Try to imagine the very worst that could happen to you and force yourself to imagine coping with this situation. When you are doing the endurance walks, imagine being lost on the hills or sustaining a broken leg. How would you then cope with bad weather?

You will never need many of these contingencies, but in simply imagining how you would cope, you are preparing yourself to meet this eventuality. Other people can be invaluable in helping you to motivate yourself. In laundering your kit, or in cooking a special meal for you, your partner can help motivate you. Friends provide that much-needed boost by simply providing the occasional lift to the gym or taking an interest in what you are trying to accomplish. Your coach at the gym will be used to working with sportsmen and women. He or she should offer encouragement, advice and the occasional compliment. They should also be prepared to offer constructive criticism when appropriate.

While nobody enjoys being criticised, think about what they are saying and see if you can use the criticism to improve your training programme. If the advice is good, it should help you to improve your performance. Success is the other great motivator; it is so easy to concentrate on the training when things are going well, but you must also be able to remain motivated and focused when the training is not going well.

The person with a well-developed character will always be able to bounce back from defeat. After a set-back, your motivation should become even stronger! The final key to motivation is enjoyment. It may not always seem possible to look forward to a hard training session, but once the session is over you should be left with that warm glow of satisfaction.

Training

Fitness training will make you more confident. It should leave you very much fitter and with a more pleasing self-image. Energy will appear to radiate from you! Knowing that you can project a self-confident image can be useful in many situations. It may enable you to control an encounter with a mugger or to deal with a tough interview with the Inland Revenue. You may well be experiencing anxiety and fear. We cannot help how we feel but we can help what we do about these feelings. Fear must be controlled and this is an important part of projecting a confident self-image. Although the real changes must take place inside you, other things can help develop a positive self-image.

The way you dress makes a statement about you. Business suits project an air of assertiveness and reliability, while less formal clothes are seen as recreational, more approachable but perhaps less reliable. Dark, loose clothing may be seen as a sign of insecurity, while people wearing bright clothing are often perceived to be confident. The way that you walk projects a particular image. An upright, purposeful stride is associated with confidence and a sense of direction. In contrast, a stooped, shuffling gait is associated with weakness, insecurity and a lack of confidence.

Tattoos and jewellery all contribute to the projected image since these often show conformity to the dress code of a minority group. Body language is something else which provides a lot of information about a person. The smiling whistler may be serenely happy or this may simply be a mask for unhappiness and a lack of confidence. It is human to advertise happiness and hide sorrow.

Fidgeting, stuttering and exaggerated movements all betray underlying feelings of disquiet and lack of self-assurance.

Eye contact, or the lack of it, can also provide interesting information about a person. A person determined to dominate the person to whom he or she is speaking will steadfastly refuse to break eye contact. Steady eye contact is invariably associated with control, aggressiveness, honesty and self-confidence, whereas the lack of eye contact is identified with a lack of confidence and dishonesty.

Body language can determine how much hassle and aggressiveness comes your way in life. Muggers and thugs learn to search for those victims less likely to put up a fight, and this type of person is often controlled and dominated by his or her partner and those in authority such as bosses, bank managers and civil servants. Be careful not to hand over control of your life to these people.

Projecting the Right Image

Real confidence must come from within. The sense of ease which comes with real self-confidence and fulfilment will determine body language and will radiate through a suit of clothes. On the other hand, no self-advertisement, no matter how well practised, will ever fully disguise a lack of confidence. Confidence springs from happiness and a sense of well-being. It is also dependent upon body image and a fitness programme can only alter your body image for the better. A diet as part of this training will also help to trim and shape your body. Feel good about your job, or work to get a better one. Strive to gain a thorough knowledge about what you do for a living. Never use bluff to disguise ignorance. Work is a central foundation of our lives; the more knowledge and experience you gain, the stronger the image you will project.

Focus

We must be mentally strong and able to focus all of our energy on what we want to achieve. Success is a mental exercise. It starts with the assertion, 'I will!' and ends with the effective projection of that willpower, directed by a good plan with realistic, achievable goals. Life is not just about succeeding; sometimes it is enough simply to overcome and survive the disappointments and set-backs. Effective survival also depends upon willpower. A long period of unemployment, for example, will demand much the same mental toughness and determination to succeed as that required by a castaway on a desert island.

The Will to Succeed

We are all born with the instinct to survive, but it can become dulled by the often monotonous routine of everyday life in a developed country.

Consequently, it becomes a skill that must be constantly re-learnt and practised. A lot of hard manual labour has been taken out of life by our modern houses, public health services and the many and various labour-saving devices which clutter our homes. Unfortunately, our comfortable lives do not prepare us for hardship; they do not necessarily make us healthier or mentally tough. Hard physical exercise within a total fitness programme goes a long way towards redressing the balance. Success, survival and sheer determination is born of willpower.

As the Irish poet Emmerson reminds us, 'Be careful about what you dream, for surely it will be yours'. Your hopes and dreams can become reality. All you have to do is provide the willpower.

Luck

Luck may favour the brave; it will certainly favour the highly motivated. If we are honest with ourselves, much 'luck' in our lives has resulted from seizing opportunities. We make our own luck. Hard work brings success and success breeds more success. There are no fairy godmothers and no point in waiting for an opportunity to walk in the door. You will be waiting a long time! You have to make it all happen.

A Sense of Humour

A sense of humour is vital to success. We all suffer many set-backs, and it is often just when you think that you are winning that disaster strikes. Humour acts as a safety valve and it helps us to put our disappointments into perspective. An SAS patrol up to their necks in swamp water and leeches will look at each other and laugh. Why not? What is the alternative? No amount of cursing or whining will alter their situation. You just have to make light of it and push on. If you can develop the ability to laugh at yourself, you will never become so angry that you blow a fuse. Remember, it is as easy to be happy in this world as it is to be miserable. If you can think positively, keep on moving forward and laugh when disaster strikes, you will eventually attain your goals.

How to Focus Your Mind

You must have a clear picture in your mind of what you want to achieve. Aim high but be realistic. If fitness is your primary goal, ask yourself why you want to become fit. If your aim is to be in an Olympic team, you will have a clear idea of the competition that you will face and the standard required to reach your goal. Make sure that all of your goals are attainable. Chart a course that will get you what you want and divide it into phases, taking one step at a time. Expect set-backs and always have contingency plans. Do not rely on other people; they will most likely let you down. Only you can help realise your ambitions. Do not make excuses for not doing things. Never leave jobs until tomorrow.

To be as good as an SAS soldier, you must be dedicated and be prepared to put in the time and effort. Nothing that is really worthwhile comes easy.

REMEMBER: When the going gets tough, the 'tough' get going.

Setting Your Goals

The best way to monitor your achievements is to use a progress chart. If you are training to achieve the very highest levels in the SAS training programme, measure your progress week by week, noting the total mileage you have covered, best personal times, average speeds and weight losses or gains. Link each challenge to some sort of reward. Recently I had an operation on my knee and I promised myself a new car when I had returned to my normal fitness. This gave me something to look forward to and helped speed my recovery. If your aim is to lose weight, try to lose $^1/_2$ kg (1 lb) per week. This will get harder as you shed that excess weight, so have a clear idea of your target weight.

If you are running to build up speed, run against your stop-watch. Time yourself over a set distance. Record your best time over the week and try to better this time next week. If your aim was, say, to run 5 km (three miles) in 18 minutes, try to maintain the same speed throughout the run. Do not run the first 1.5 km (one mile) in six minutes, the next in eight minutes and the last 1.5 km (one mile) in ten minutes. If you cover a 5-km (three-mile) course in 24 minutes, aim to run each 1.5 km (one mile) in eight minutes. Now try to shave a minute off each 1.5 km (one mile). Your next target will be to run each 1.5 km (one mile) in seven minutes and 30 seconds. This is by far the easiest way to attain your objective.

If body-building is your aim, then take my advice and do not try to keep up with your companions in the gym. Do not worry if they are lifting heavier weights than you. They may have bigger builds and may need the heavier weights just to gain the same benefits.

Depression

Some days are definitely better than others. You can feel terrific on Monday, but by Wednesday everything seems to be an effort. There can be many reasons for your change of mood. You may be sleeping badly, there may be problems at work or you may have picked up a mild dose of the flu. The weather can be responsible for our mood swings. We always feel better when the sun is shining. Many people become a little depressed in winter or during long spells of bad weather.

A change in pace or lifestyle can help restore our sense of humour and our positive outlook on life. Exercise is another potent defence against depression, but even your training programme can become a struggle. Do not despair or give up! Change your programme and place the emphasis on different activities. A change can be as good as a rest. When you return to the original programme after a week or so, you will see remarkable progress.

Above all, do not stop training. Hard physical training can alter the body chemistry responsible for depression and can offer a sense of achievement and fulfilment. Your SAS training programme should become part of your overall effort to achieve your goals. Realistic, attainable goals in life are another potent defence against depression.

Finally, always try to look on the bright side of life and count your blessings. There are many, many people worse off than yourself.

Fear

Fear is another obstacle we must all face and overcome. It can take many forms, ranging from the mild anxiety we all feel before an important interview, to an overwhelming sense of panic which can cripple your life. Firstly, do not be ashamed of fear. It is a natural 'fight or flight' response that comes into play when we perceive a threat, be it real or imagined. It is just unfortunate that, while the sudden jolt of adrenalin was a real life-saver for our prehistoric ancestors, it may have outlived its usefulness.

In much of everyday life, this primitive defence reaction is both inconvenient and inappropriate. Here is some advice for overcoming fear.

- Try to put your problems into perspective. It has been said that 'nothing matters much and very little matters much at all'. Very few incidents or decisions have a lasting effect on our lives.
- Become philosophical about life. We cannot double-guess life. It is a constant cycle of joy and sorrow, success and defeat, frustration and achievement. We worry needlessly about a whole range of life problems. We may worry about getting a particular job but, even if we are unsuccessful, another job will come along. With hindsight, we can remember many instances, perceived at the time as defeats, that actually changed our lives for the better. Several years ago, a friend of mine was crushed when he lost his job. He worked in a large financial institution in London which was taken over by Arab interests. The bank was to move to the Gulf and he was not selected to join the new 'stream-lined team'. At the time it seemed to be the end of all of his hopes and aspirations and the future looked very uncertain. After eight months unemployment, he found another job which, in providing much more leisure time, changed his life for the better. One morning he opened the paper to discover that his friends who had kept their jobs with the bank and had moved to Kuwait had been taken prisoner by the Iraqi Army.
- Imagine yourself confronting a situation that makes you feel anxious. Play it through in your mind and imagine getting the better of the situation. We all experience fear; some of us are just more practised at coping with it or disguising it.
- Be a professional. Both the professional entertainer waiting to go on stage and the novice faced with delivering a talk in front of an audience will experience anxiety. The major difference is that the professional says to him or herself, 'This is my job, it is how I want to spend my life. I will master my fear because it is part of the job'. We can all strive for professionalism in everything that we try to accomplish.
- Learn to control the urge to panic. Panic is the most destructive of our emotions. It should never be tolerated. Breathing exercises can help switch off the effects of that dreadful surge of adrenalin. A Japanese psychiatrist found the following exercise very successful in helping his patients cope with panic. It can be used in every situation.

  1 Stand or sit upright.
  2 Take a deep breath through the mouth, filling your lungs.
  3 Exhale very slowly through the nose. Imagine that you are holding a feather in front of your nose and exhale so gently that the 'feather' remains perfectly still.

- Confidence is the greatest enemy of fear and panic. Use your SAS training programme to help attain your goals and develop that wonderful sense of achievement. Achievement, fulfilment and inner happiness are the well-spring of confidence.

CHAPTER FIFTEEN
Pressure at Work

In our everyday lives, we find ourselves subject to a number of pressures. Some are real, some imagined, and some are self-inflicted or, at the very least, avoidable. Problems with punctuality are self-inflicted. Some people make a habit of being late; they never allow themselves enough time to get to appointments or they manage their available time poorly.

These are symptoms of poor time management. When people use the excuse 'Oh, I haven't got time', what they really mean is that they are too lazy to sort themselves out. One of the first lessons taught by the SAS is good time management. SAS operations rely on precise time-keeping. Squadrons are expected to move to anywhere in the world with just a few hours' notice. Patrols are expected to keep to their operational schedules; their work is dangerous but the risks can be reduced by precise timing. An operational rendezvous may remain 'open' for only five minutes each side of the allotted time. Here is my prescription for good time-keeping:

♦ Rise when the alarm clock rings. Resist the temptation to stay in bed.
♦ Remember the six 'P's: Prior Planning Prevents a Piss-Poor Performance.

Plan Your Day
Your plan should contain generous allowances for heavy traffic or difficulties in finding a parking place.

Careful preparation is another hallmark of SAS operations. Like the SAS soldier, prepare for tomorrow today. Make sure the car has a full tank of petrol. It is easy to forget where we have left things when we are in a hurry. Have a place for everything and stick to it. Hang up your keys where they cannot be misplaced.

If you are arranging to meet somebody in a crowded place, choose a clearly identifiable meeting point. If you are meeting a stranger, make sure that you can identify each other. Check that you have all of your paper-work and mentally run through tomorrow's events. Make sure that you have everything you will need such as money, contact telephone numbers, tickets and spare change for parking meters.

People are not always punctual and can fail to turn up on time for meetings for a whole range of reasons. Make sure that they know how to contact you if they are unexpectedly delayed.

Allow yourself a minimum of 15 minutes to find a place to park the car, make sure that you are in the right building, use the toilet and run a comb through your hair.

Before Taking the Job

Choose your place of work carefully. Both before and after your interview, look very carefully at the firm and its work place. Talk to some of the staff and try to ascertain whether the firm are good employers and whether there are any local problems. Is there a high annual staff turnover? This may indicate that staff are expected to attain impossible targets. Ask the existing staff how often they are expected to take work home or work weekends. Some highly paid sales and managerial firms have staff turnover rates as high as 25 per cent per annum.

A firm which loses one person in four every year, is likely to be in many ways a 'hostile environment'. If you are nevertheless tempted to take the job, ask yourself the question: Am I prepared to die for this firm? Stress directly contributes to a range of fatal diseases. In addition, one in four people will experience some sort of psychiatric complaint during the course of their lives. Many psychiatric illnesses are either caused or precipitated by high levels of stress.

Devotion Beyond the Call of Duty?

If you find yourself working most evenings and weekends, you are implicitly sacrificing family members, friends and what could have been a fascinating and fulfilling life. You should also ask yourself if you are really suited for the job for which you are applying. Can you ride out the stress of coping with an unfamiliar work place and rise to the challenge? The first three to six months in a job are usually the most stressful. Do not forget that tasks that at first seem very complex, after practice and repetition, can almost appear to be child's play.

Assessing Your Future Colleagues and Work Enviroment

Are your colleagues the sort of people with whom you can rub along and have some laughs? After all, you are intending to spend a large proportion of your life with these people. What is the firm's policy on smoking? Staff should not be expected to inhale other people's cigarette smoke. Stress is an inherent part of all jobs but, for the most part, it should be that enjoyable form of pressure which comes from solving problems and meeting your work targets. Today, most managers accept that a healthy work environment and good managerial practices make for a contented work force, higher productivity and a low absentee rate. Other firms behave as though they were still living in the nineteenth century. Some treat their employees like children. Others treat their staff as though they were disposable. You can play an important role in minimising stress by choosing your job carefully.

Controlling the Stress in Your Life

Stress is a part of everyday life. Too little stress can be as bad as too much. As anyone who has experienced a long period of unemployment knows, work and its associated stresses gives our lives a structure and a sense of fulfilment. The trick is to control the stress. The day's stress can start with the rush hour and heavy traffic. You can, of course, leave that little bit earlier to avoid the worst of the traffic. Be courteous. Smile at other road users. Make a point of stopping to allow traffic to leave side roads. Give pedestrians priority, particularly at crossings. What goes around comes around.

We all have the opportunity to help shape the sort of world in which we would like to live. If you are faced with a long drive, put some relaxing music on the tape deck. Take a colleague to work and take turns at driving. Investigate alternative routes along minor roads. The drive may be longer but a lot more pleasant. Public transport can be more stressful than busy roads. If you are faced with standing, make a space for yourself.

Stand with your arms bent and elbows out to the side. Try to stay in the centre of crowds getting on and off trains and buses. As far as possible maintain your own space. Wear stout, comfortable shoes. Make sure that your chair at the office is comfortable.

Redundancy is an ever-present danger in modern life. You can do little about hostile take-overs and financial collapse but you can try to ensure that you are not the first to be sacked. Be a diligent worker. Strive to meet your deadlines, sales figures or delivery dates. Individual competition within an office can be self-defeating for everyone. Try to persuade your fellow workers to co-operate and work together. Always be prepared to lend somebody else a hand. Show leadership to the younger and newer members of the team. Working within friendly groups helps buffer individuals from stress.

Recognising Stress

At some point in our lives, most of us will exhibit some symptoms of stress. It is important to recognise these little distress signals and either work to reduce the stress in our lives or seek medical advice. The symptoms of stress can include:

Loss of appetite
Teeth grinding, nail biting and playing with hair
Falling asleep in front of the television or in meetings
An inability to drop off to sleep or waking too early
Persistent headaches
Feelings of tiredness and a lack of interest in life
Sweating and swimming head
Loss of confidence in yourself
Difficulty in making decisions
Exaggerated response to sudden loud noise
Diarrhoea and nausea
A marked increase in alcohol or tobacco consumption
Uncharacteristic forgetfulness

The following symptoms of anxiety and panic require prompt medical attention and intervention.

Emotional Vulnerability: The person feels like crying and when they cry, they cannot seem to stop.

Panic Attacks: Shallow, rapid breathing; inability to think, rapid pulse rate, sweating and feelings of impending disaster. The 'fight or flight' response has switched over entirely to 'flight'.

Unreasonable Fear: The person is in a constant state of fear.

Agoraphobia: This can take the form of a fear of open spaces but often presents as a fear of crowds, shopping or even leaving the house. This is simply a defence reaction to overwhelming stress in which the person attempts to avoid all the normal forms of stress.

Obsessions: Obessions often occur as distinct illnesses, but a person under stress can also develop obsessions. The stressed housewife feels an overwhelming desire to return home to check that, for example, she has turned off the cooker. The stressed executive constantly checks to ensure that his or her papers are in his or her briefcase.

Dealing with Stress

The first problem is recognising that you are stressed. Hard-working, ambitious people who take on great responsibilities accept a lot of stress in their lives. Much of this is enjoyable but circumstances can change and they can find themselves 'burdened' with additional stress. They are often the last people to admit that something is wrong. Once a person has recognised that he or she is under pressure, steps must be taken to reduce stress.

- A lot of additional stressful work can be delegated to employees and other family members.
- Talk about your problems to your partner and close friends. Psychiatrists and psychologists often just fill the role of 'professional listeners'. The stressed individual is often over-joyed to discover a close friend who has had to cope with many of the same problems.
- Accept that you are just as human and vulnerable as anyone else in the world. Stress is common. People experiencing the symptoms of stress and anxiety often fearfully confess to their doctor that they are 'going mad'. They are not going mad and they are not alone. Stress-related illness is extremely common.
- Take a holiday or some time off. Make sure that your weekends are spent doing what you want to do. Move at a slower pace; everyday life was not meant to be a competitive sport. Take time to stop and talk to friends and acquaintances. Do not superimpose a schedule on your leisure time. Do not try to achieve the impossible in a day.
- Avoid the 'quick fixes'. Do not try to mask your feelings with alcohol.

The problems will still be there tomorrow, only now you will have to cope with the hangover as well. Tranquillisers and sleeping pills are very good at providing the user with a 'chemical holiday', but they should only be used for short periods.

- Make space for yourself. Learn to say 'no'. Demand some private space and leisure time. This may mean buying an answer-machine or turning off the telephone at weekends. It may mean resisting the temptation to crowd your diary with appointments. Place another person between yourself and the incessant clamour for your attention.
- Forget the macho nonsense. A person crumpling under stress is often afflicted with feelings of shame and inadequacy. There is no shame in suffering from stress. Every single living soul has their breaking point and in every case it will be different. The symptoms of stress are Nature's distress signal. Read the signal correctly; start to identify and either change or eliminate the stressful areas of your life.
- Take a hard look at your life. There is much in our lives that we can change. The problem is that we naturally fear change. Take a pen and paper and on one side of the paper list all the problems in your life which are stressing you. On the other side of the paper force yourself to list possible solutions. S

SAS Relaxation Exercises

Exercises can help you relax and find an inner peace. We were taught this one in the Regiment and it never fails to work:

1 Stand erect, feet shoulder-width apart. Hold your arms out, palms upward and elbows tucked into the body.
2 Close your eyes and breathe in through your mouth. Hold your breath for the count of five and tense your body. Lock your legs. Strain your hands to make fists and draw your arms back to your waist.
3 Release your breath as you push your arms forward and allow your whole body to relax.
4 As you repeat this exercise, imagine yourself in a room filled with white light. As you breathe in, you will inhale this beautiful light. As you exhale, all the anger and frustrations leave your body like a black cloud. Continue with the exercise until you can imagine your body filled with the light.

CHAPTER SIXTEEN
Facing Danger

SAS soldiers will often find themselves in dangerous situations, and part of their training teaches them to recognise threats and make the correct decision as to what to do about them. They are taught to look for their enemies' strengths and weaknesses and formulate a course of action. This chapter will teach you how to assess people in various situations and predict their responses. The most dangerous situation in which you will ever find yourself will probably be those rare instances when you are faced with a violent confrontation. The most common and yet most difficult situations that you will encounter will be having to deal with agressive salesmen or onerous officials. In all of these situations, the ability to correctly interpret 'body language' will give you a hidden advantage.

Physical Threats
Most incidents involving physical violence can be avoided. Self-defence begins with recognising threats and potentially dangerous situations and taking action to avoid them.

Stay Alert: In the SAS, we are taught to scan the ground ahead. With practice this becomes second nature.

First scan the ground immediately ahead of you, from right to left. Immediately raise your eyes and begin another sweep a little higher than the first. Finally, your gaze should sweep across the middle and far distance.

Rapid scanning covers a lot of ground with very little effort. If during a sweep you notice something suspicious or odd, look closely until you can decide whether it is just something unusual, for example an open door, a group of kids loitering on a street corner, a couple of down-and-outs on a bench, or a possible threat such as a figure in a darkened doorway, a group of youths blocking the pavement, youths who are paying you a lot of attention or aggressive drunks on a bench.

Check Your Back: On SAS patrols, it is the job of the 'rear scout' or the last man to check for danger behind the patrol. In the street, this means much more than just occasionally turning around to check behind you. Streets are full of totally innocent people going about their business. The sudden appearance behind you of a scruffy individual in a darkened street may seem threatening but this may simply be your perception of the situation. **Take Evasive Action:** Detour along an alternative route and see if he continues to follow you. The chances are that he is innocent.

Work Out An Escape Route: Just in case, look for an immediate place of safety, such as shops, other people or a house where the occupants are obviously at home. Escape routes are another SAS technique which will help you avoid confrontation. No matter where you find yourself, plan an escape route. Really, this is just common sense. The crew of a commercial aircraft or ferry are required by law to ensure that all the passengers are informed of the whereabouts of emergency exits. In hotels, cinemas and other public buildings you should locate the fire exits or service doors for yourself. Disasters only happen rarely, but when they do, those first few precious minutes can make the difference between living and dying.

Taking Precautions

Route planning is about avoiding areas where you can be easily ambushed. Where possible, avoid open ground, poorly lit streets, alleys, under-passes, and areas of town known for violence. Stay on well-used thoroughfares and mingle with crowds. As far as your personal protection is concerned, other people provide camouflage, concealment and are a potential source of help. Major routes also provide a variety of escape routes such as shops, police stations, cinemas and public houses where you can obtain help.

To minimise the risk to your safety, behave confidently and purposefully. Walk with your head up and keep your hands free. Avoid eye contact with strangers. Youths, particularly, may take eye-contact as a challenge to their 'respect', while the profiles of many violent men mark them as unusually paranoid. Glance in their direction and then look away. Never look down at the ground since this is a very submissive gesture. If in some crowded place such as a train or a pub you find that somebody is staring at you, turn your body away from the pest, fixing your gaze in the middle distance, while keeping them in your peripheral vision. This avoids confrontation, allows you to keep an eye on them and forces them into a game which they cannot win! Bags and cases mark you as a target for muggers. When carrying a case or bag in the street, transfer it to the inside shoulder or hand and walk close to the wall. Force people to walk around you on the outside.

Carry an old wallet crammed with paper cut to the same size as bank notes. Equally, an old purse can be filled with foreign coins or metal washers. If confronted by a mugger, quickly hand over the 'dummy' wallet or purse. He will probably cover a considerable distance before checking his haul! Wear a stout but comfortable pair of lace-up shoes so that you can make a quick get-away.

Criminals, particularly those who abuse drugs, cigarettes and alcohol are not exactly 'track star' material and can be easily out-distanced by the young and vigorous. Stout shoes also bring a little something extra to a good kick, if you find yourself in a tight corner. If feeling particularly threatened, you might consider carrying a walking stick or umbrella to fend off an assaillant. Loose, comfortable clothes are less restricting in a confrontation.

The Confrontation

If confronted by an aggressive or angry person, try and stay calm. If you panic, you simply place yourself at your attacker's mercy. Slow, regular breathing will help control your emotions. Look for escape routes but, above all, remember your self-defence training.

Self-defence in the gym and in the street begins with the concept of 'personal space'. Imagine you are standing in the centre of a circle with a diameter of just over 1 m (4 ft). This is your personal space. By the very term 'self-defence', we understand that the person defending themselves will not attack first. The defender retains a considerable advantage because, to attack you, your assailant will have to enter your personal space. In making the first move, your attacker enters an area of space protected by your arm and leg strikes. Stand in a disguised guarding position. Your body should be side-on to your attacker (it makes less of a target). Your arms and hands should be ready for action and yet guarding the head and ribs. Your right leg (if you favour the right side of your body) should be slightly behind your left leg and ready to launch a powerful kick if necessary!

Index